Cardiac Pacing and Monitoring - New Methods, Modern Devices

Edited by Mart Min

Published in London, United Kingdom

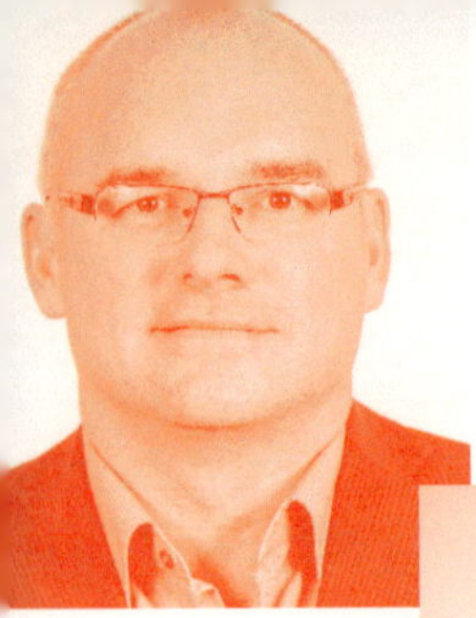
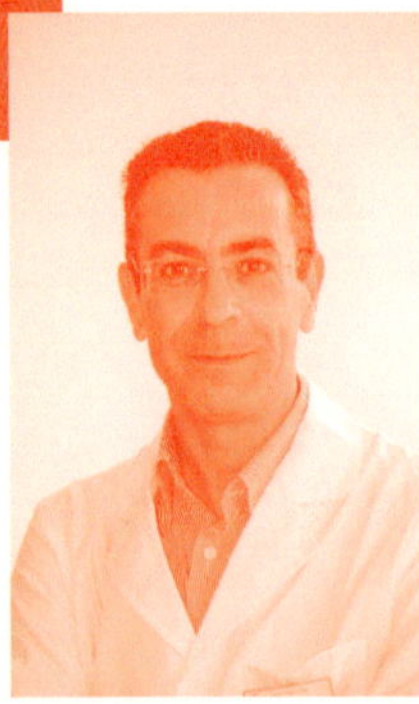
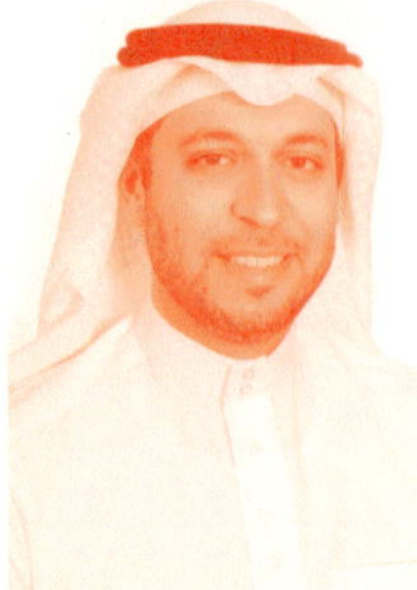
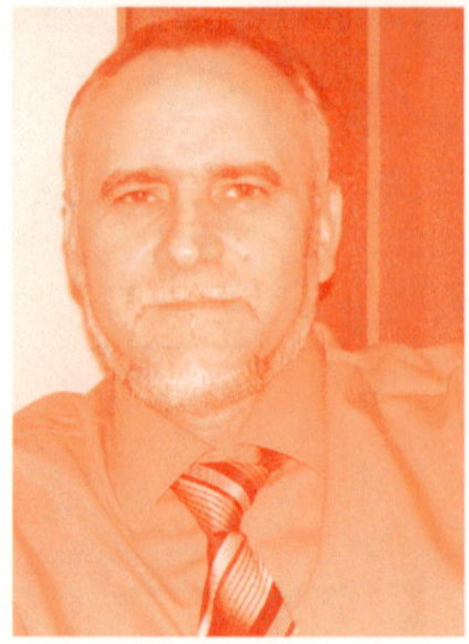
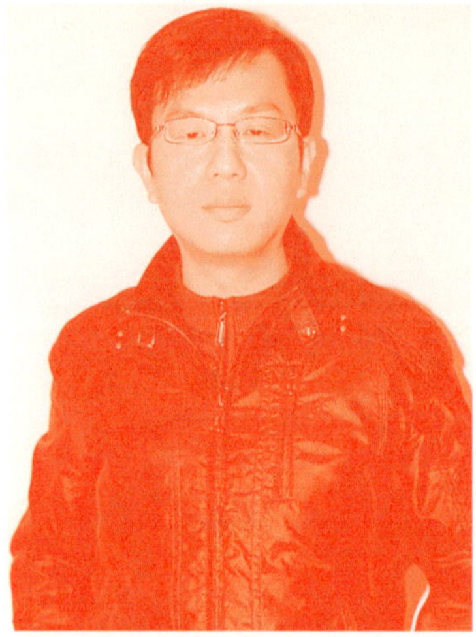
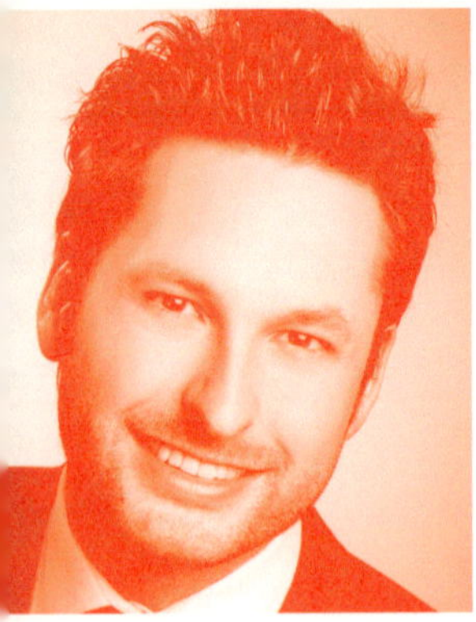
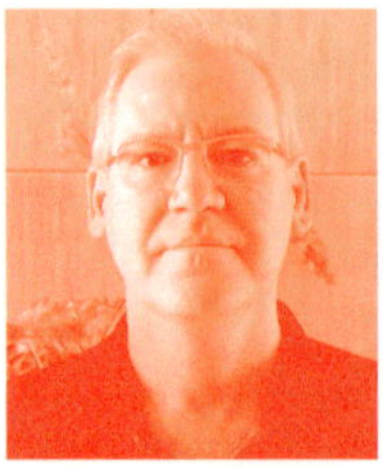

IntechOpen

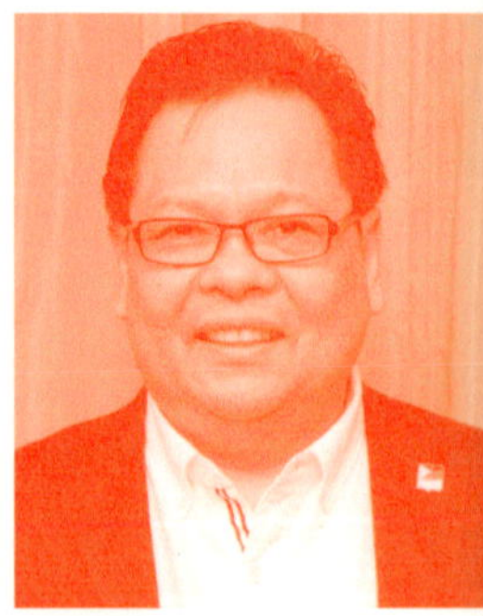
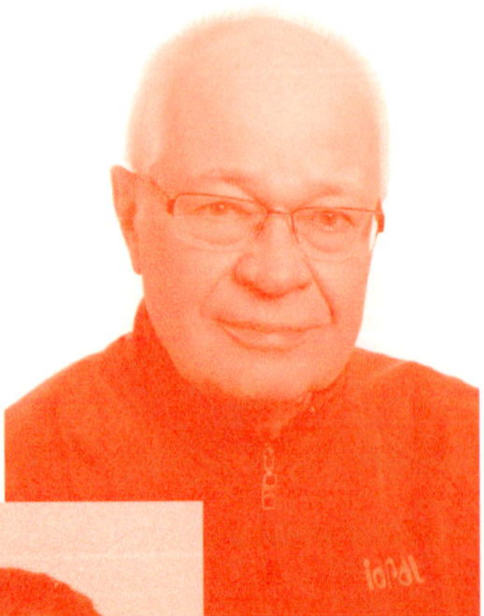
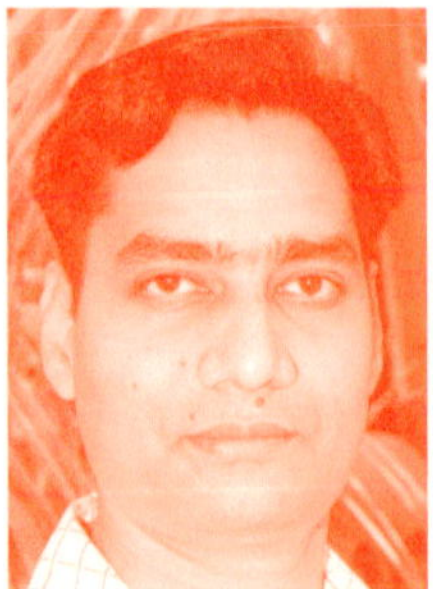
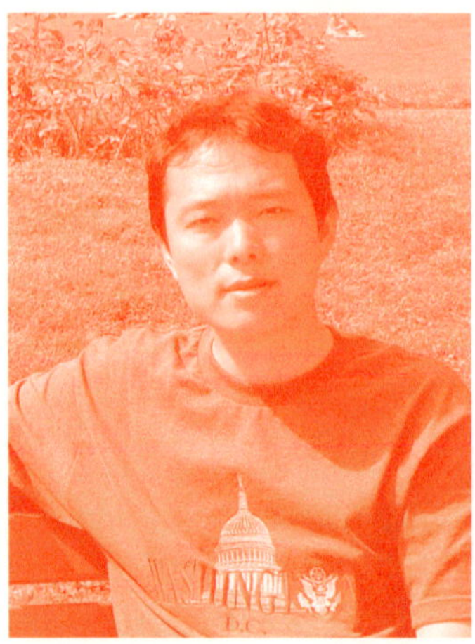
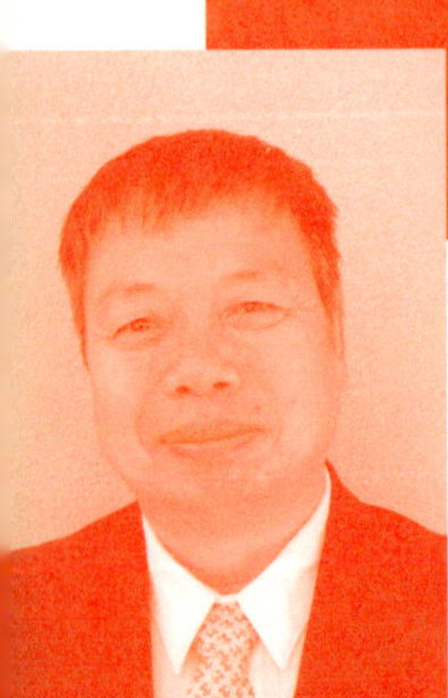
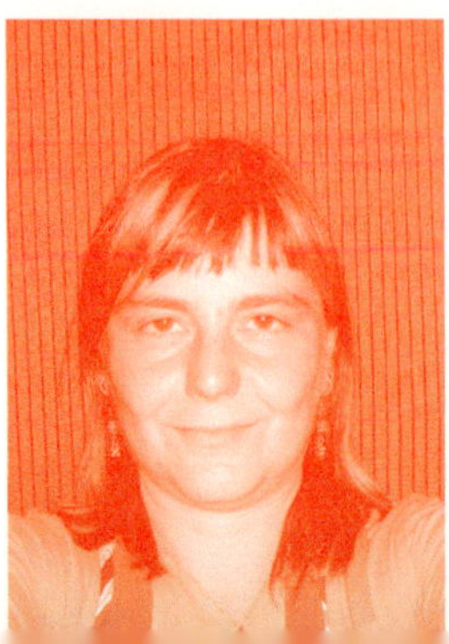

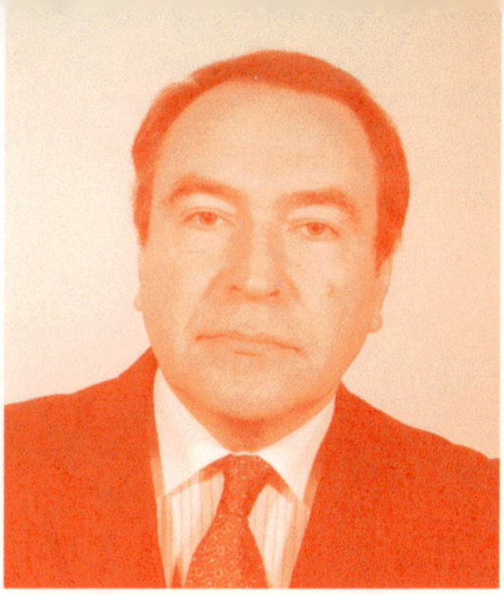
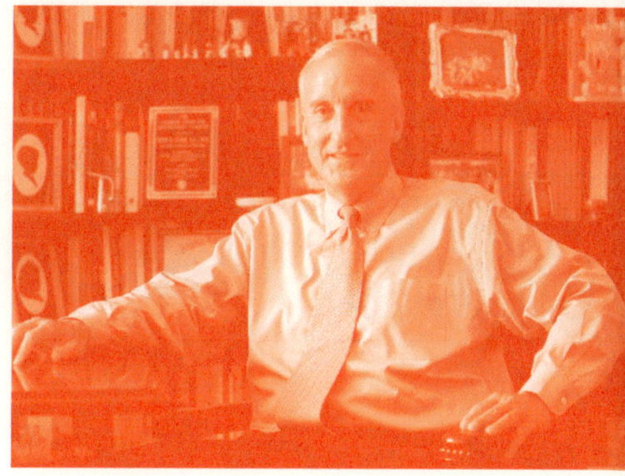
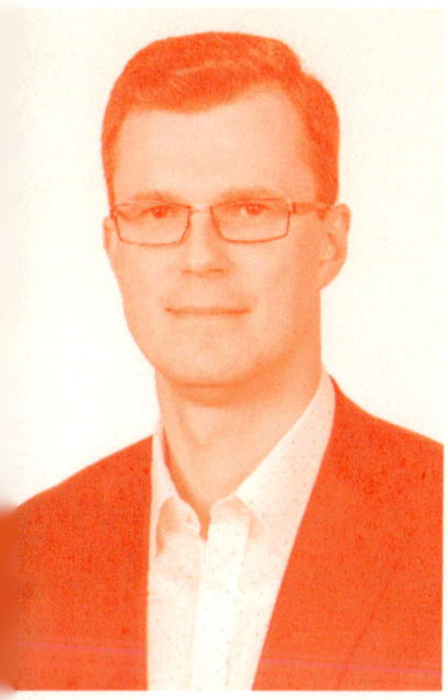
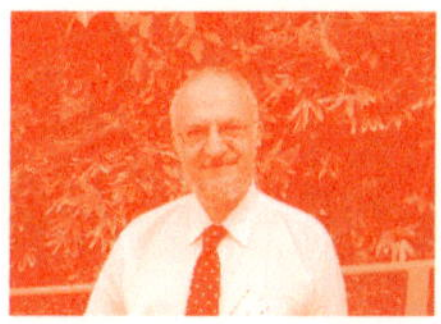
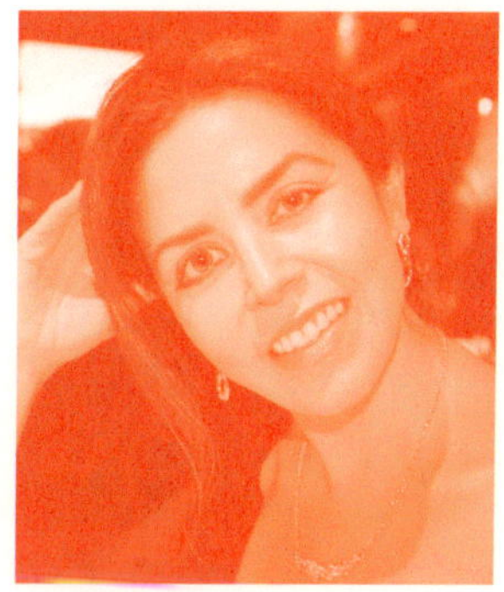

Supporting open minds since 2005

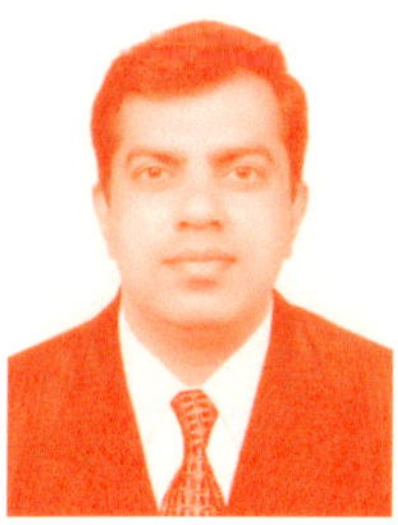
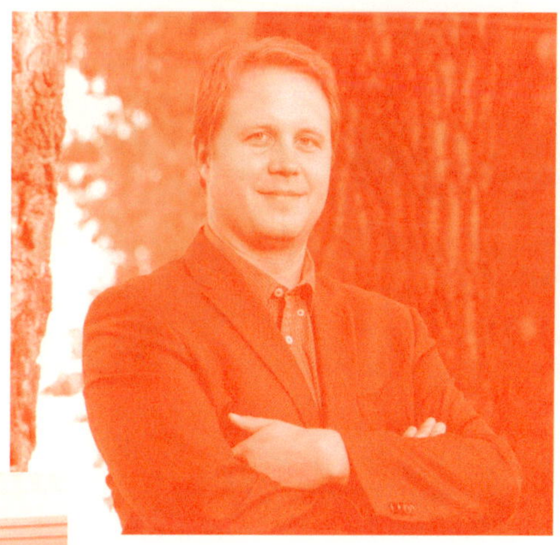
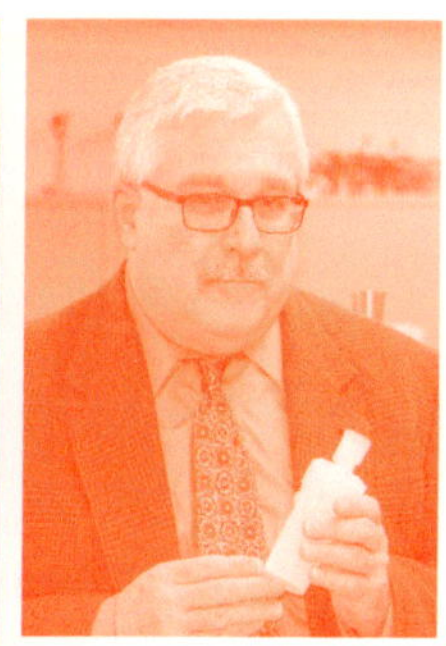
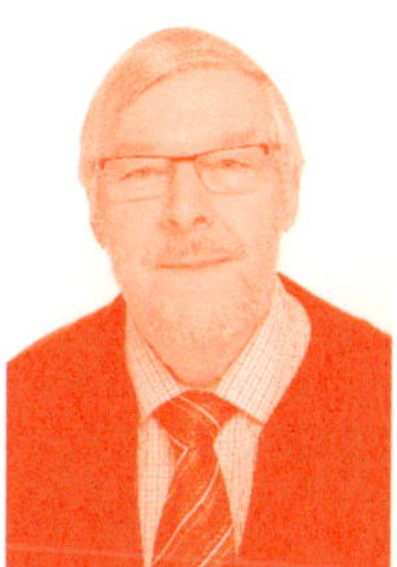
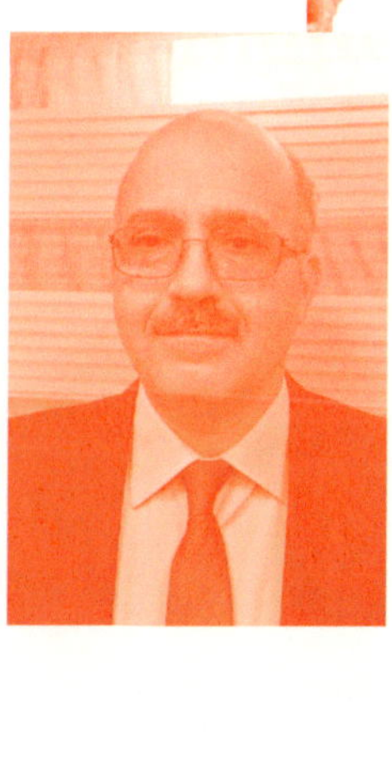
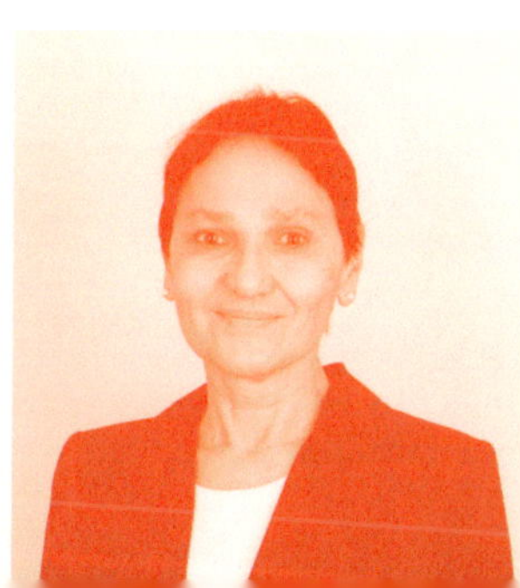
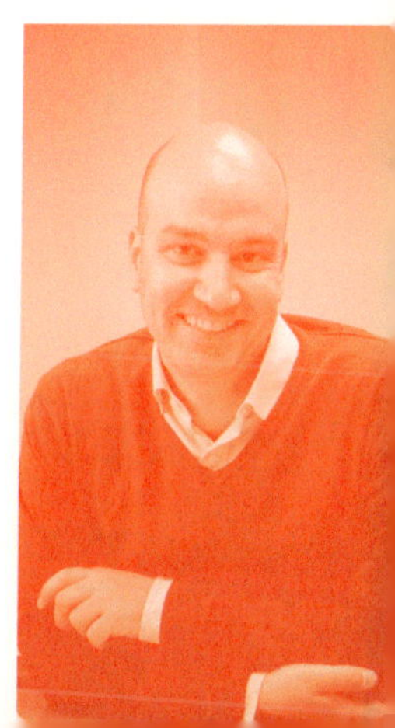

Cardiac Pacing and Monitoring - New Methods, Modern Devices
http://dx.doi.org/10.5772/intechopen.73811
Edited by Mart Min

Contributors
Gustav Mattsson, Ida Åberg, Peter Michael Magnusson, Jo Ann LeQuang, Joseph Pergolizzi, Joseph V. Pergolizzi, Jr., Magnus Samuelsson, Hani Anabi, Mart Min

First published in London, United Kingdom, 2019 by IntechOpen
IntechOpen is the global imprint of INTECHOPEN LIMITED, registered in England and Wales, registration number: 11086078, The Shard, 25th floor, 32 London Bridge Street
London, SE19SG - United Kingdom
Printed in Croatia

British Library Cataloguing-in-Publication Data
A catalogue record for this book is available from the British Library

Additional hard copies can be obtained from orders@intechopen.com

Cardiac Pacing and Monitoring - New Methods, Modern Devices
Edited by Mart Min
p. cm.
Print ISBN 978-1-83880-179-3
Online ISBN 978-1-83880-180-9

For EU product safety concerns:
IN TECH d.o.o., Prolaz Marije Krucifikse Kozulić 3, 51000 Rijeka, Croatia, info@intechopen.com or visit our website at intechopen.com.

Meet the editor

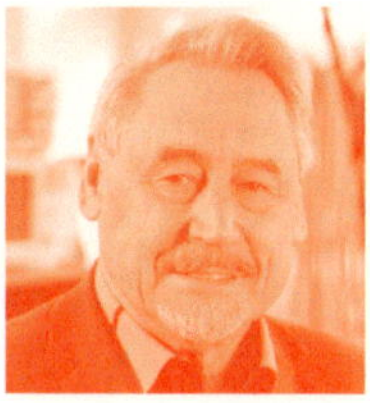

Dr. Mart Min has been a professor and leading scientist at Thomas Johann Seebeck Department of Electronics, Tallinn University of Technology, Estonia, since 1992. He received his PhD degree in Measurement Science from Kiev Polytechnic, Ukraine, in 1984. Between 1992 and 1993, he was with the Technical University and the Bundeswehr University in Munich, Germany. Between 2007 and 2010, Dr. Min worked at the Institute of Bioprocessing and Analytical Measurement Techniques, Germany. His interests include sensing and processing of biological signals and developing pacemakers for St. Jude Medical (USA). He has hundreds of publications and tens of patents in the field. Dr. Min is a senior member of the IEEE EMB Society. He retired from his professor emeritus position in 2017 but continues research in medical electronics.

Contents

Preface XI

Chapter 1 1
Introductory Chapter: From Basic Foundations to Future Developments
by Mart Min

Chapter 2 9
Clinical Indications for Therapeutic Cardiac Devices
by Ida Åberg, Gustav Mattsson and Peter Magnusson

Chapter 3 31
The Subcutaneous Implantable Cardioverter-Defibrillator
by Peter Magnusson, Joseph V. Pergolizzi and Jo Ann LeQuang

Chapter 4 47
Leadless Pacemakers
by Peter Magnusson, Joseph V. Pergolizzi Jr and Jo Ann LeQuang

Chapter 5 71
Atrial Fibrillation and the Role of Thumb ECGs
by Peter Magnusson, Magnus Samuelsson, Joseph V. Pergolizzi Jr, Hani Annabi and Jo Ann LeQuang

Preface

Clinical usage of artificial pacing with the aid of implantable devices dates back to 1958, when battery-powered cardiac pacemakers became available. Modern implantable pacemakers are complex self-controlled electronic devices operating 10–12 years continuously without battery exchange. Although the design of devices is not a primary topic of this book, their development has been addressed through a historical overview from the late 1950s up until the variety of modern-day equipment.

Most attention is paid to the selection of pacing and monitoring devices for implementation in different medical situations. The discussion is oriented toward specifying the clinical indications for implanting the most appropriate cardiac device from the selection of suitable equipment.

Indications for using the most appropriate models of cardiac pacemakers, cardiac resynchronization therapy devices, and implantable cardioverter defibrillators (ICDs) are of interest, paying special attention to the leadless versions of the devices. The contraindications of patients' different health conditions are taken into account carefully. Placing of leads and pacing electrodes has been treated soundly, but particular attention is paid to using leadless devices. For example, the subcutaneous ICD obviates the need for trouble-making transvenous leads and leadless pacemakers are entirely implantable into the right ventricle. Finally, applications of user-friendly wearable devices for the detection and analyses of atrial arrhythmia are discussed.

The authors have derived useful information from both their own clinical practice and the experiences of their close colleagues. Practical knowledge and scientific basics related to pragmatic issues are the most valuable assets of this book.

Mart Min
Tallinn University of Technology,
Estonia

Chapter 1

Introductory Chapter: From Basic Foundations to Future Developments

Mart Min

1. Early pacemakers

Dr. Rune Elmqvist (1906–1996), a physician working for the Swedish company Elema-Schönander (later a part of Siemens) as an engineer, developed the first implantable pacemaker. Dr. Elmqvist developed the device in cooperation with Åke Senning (1915–2000), a senior physician and cardiac surgeon at the Hospital of Karolinska Institute in Solna near Stockholm [1]. Their first patient, Arne Larsson (1915–2001), underwent secret emergency surgery to implant his first pacemaker on October 8, 1958, just in the middle of his lifetime. The role of his wife Else-Marie was important. She persuaded the scientists to make the surgery, though they strongly refused, initially. Finally, it was an officially unacceptable prank, made under the pressure of female power! Later Arne Larsson went on to receive more than 20 pacemakers in the 43 years following the first implantation.

The pacemaker contained a single transistor-based blocking pulse oscillator which delivered pacing impulses at an amplitude of 2 V and a pulse width of 1.5 ms through a transistor buffer. The frequency of pulse sequence was set to have a constant rate pacing of 70 beats per minute. The energy utilized by a totally two-transistor electronic circuit from a nickel-cadmium battery was minimal since Elmqvist managed to obtain a few of the first silicon transistors produced by Texas Instruments, USA. Recharging of the battery once a week for 12 h was accomplished inductively by a 150 kHz radio frequency current generated externally.

Dr. Elmqvist produced two of such handmade units encapsulated in a new epoxy resin (Araldite), which had excellent biocompatibility. He used a shoe polish can from Kiwi with a diameter 55 mm and thickness of 16 mm as a mold.

After being a young trainee of Dr. Åke Senning in Sweden, Dr. Orestes Fiandra (later founder of the company CCC del Uruguay, now Integer) implanted a pacemaker designed by Dr. Rune Elmqvist and produced by Elema-Schönander (Sweden), in Uruguay on February 2, 1960, together with Dr. Roberto Rubio.

In parallel, Earl E. Bakken (1914–2018), an electrical engineer and co-founder of the company Medtronic in 1949 in Minneapolis, USA, made a transistor-based blocking oscillator for the first battery-operated wearable pacemaker (1957). Famous doctor C. Walton Lillehei (1918–1999) from the University of Minnesota, "the father of open chest surgery," took the device into medical use in 1958. This pacemaker became known as the Medtronic Cardiac Pacemaker 5800 (produced in 1958). The chosen pacemaker output was a 2 ms square wave, variable in amplitude from 1 to 20 mA into a 1000 Ω load, which gives from 1 to 20 V. The pacing rate was variable from 60 to 180 pulses per minute. Meanwhile, Dr. Lillehei and his co-workers developed the myocardial wire (1957) for the implanting of pacemakers:

IntechOpen

a braided stainless steel wire in a Teflon sleeve implemented directly into the myocardium, while the other end was connected to the pacemaker via stab incision. To close the electrical circuit, a common (neutral) large area electrode was buried under the skin. As a result, only 1.5 V is needed for effective pacing. Meanwhile (1958), a transvenous catheter electrode was introduced fluoroscopically via the basilic vein into the right ventricle. Medtronic Inc. continues production of the cardiac rhythm devices being nowadays the largest medical technology company in the world.

At about the same time, in 1958, Mr. Wilson Greatbatch (1919–2011) was working on the recording of tachycardias. He recognized that the low-level electrical current could power the implantable pacemaker and drive a human heart. Mr. Greatbatch asked Dr. William Chardack (1915–2006), chief of surgery at Buffalo's Veterans Hospital, and surgeon Dr. Andrew Gage to test a mercury battery-powered implantable pacemaker at the hospital's animal lab. The design was proven to work.

In 1960, Dr. Chardack successfully implanted the device in a 77-year-old man, who lived for 2 years before dying of unrelated causes. Later Medtronic Inc. owned the Chardack-Greatbatch pacemaker [2]. Mr. Greatbatch invented also the lithium battery for pacemakers [3] and formed a company Wilson Greatbatch Ltd. for the production of these batteries. The company continues to save the lives of patients worldwide as a part of Integer Holdings Corporation. Modern batteries can work 10–12 years continuously in nowadays pacemakers.

2. Demand pacemaker

The next big step was invention of the demand pacemaker by Barouh V. Berkovits [4]. The early pacemakers generated pacing pulses continuously at a preset constant frequency/rate regardless of any spontaneous activity of the heart, that is, whether the natural pacemaker in the heart beats or not. The competition of two pacing sources took place, and, as a result, arrhythmias and/or ventricular fibrillation provoked making normal heart work impossible. The demand pacemaker has sensing electronics for the detecting of natural pacing. The artificial pacing switched off when the natural one works. The demand pacemaker contains the first implantable cardiac monitor inside.

3. Physiological pacing

One more step leads us to physiological pacing introduced with implementation of the dual-chamber pacemaker having the electrodes for synchronized pacing and exact timing in both the right atrium and right ventricle. This pacemaker senses the natural activity of atrium and ventricle separately. The aim is to define, whether, and in which compartment – in atrium, ventricle or in both – the artificial pacing is required at certain moments to achieve the best mimicking of natural heart work, see the US Patent by Berkovits [5]. However, the latest investigation shows that achieving adequate physiological pacing still remains problematic even nowadays, 50 years later.

Attempts to achieve left ventricle (LV) pacing are introduced for getting more exact physiological pacing. There is still no way to move the pacing electrodes directly into the left ventricle because of too high blood pressure delivered there. Therefore, different indirect pacing ways were introduced. First, left ventricle septal pacing shows to be promising in restoring the pumping performance. Then, endocardial and epicardial LV pacing modes are introduced, where endocardial stimulation appears to be more physiological and less problematic than epicardial activation.

Cardiac resynchronization therapy (CRT) using biventricular (BIV) pacing has proved its effectiveness to correct myocardial asynchrony [6] and improve clinical status of patients with severe congestive heart failure (CHF). Multipolar LV leads for multisite pacing have recently become available for biventricular pacing [7].

4. Rate-responsive pacing

While earlier pacemakers have a predetermined pacing rate, set to fixed "optimal" value, rate-responsive adaptive pacemakers speed up or slow down your heart rate depending on metabolic demand of your body. Modern rate-responsive pacemakers are capable of adapting to a wide range of sensors information relating to physiological needs depending on physical activity of the patient. The first proposal to introduce the adaption of pacing rate to respiratory parameters was made in 1967 already [8], but real implementation of rate-responsive pacing began in the early 1980s [9].

Rate-responsive pacemakers use a physiologic sensor in the cardiac monitor embedded into the pacemaker to adjust the pacing rate according to the physiologic needs of the patient, which is proportional to his/her metabolic demand. The latter is the response to an oxygen debt.

It should ideally operate in a closed-loop system, making rate-adaptive pacing insensitive to not heart-related inputs. Finally, dedicated sensors should avoid undesirable over pacing. Safety operation needs reliable electronics and complex programming.

4.1 Sensing and monitoring

Different parameters have been investigated for the regulating of pacing rate: oxygen saturation, venous pH, QT interval, body motion, respiratory rate, stroke volume, central venous temperature, minute ventilation, peak endocardial acceleration, and changes of the right ventricular impedance during the cardiac cycle (closed-loop stimulation). Clinical studies have outlined advantages and limitations of the different sensed parameters; only some of these are still used in sensor technology.

Only some of these sensing principles are in practical use; nowadays, all of which are unable to recognize the oxygen debt directly.

Activity sensors are older and more widely used. The principle of work of these sensors bases on the relationship between the physical activity and the corresponding heart rate. Activity may be acknowledged either (1) by a piezoelectric crystal, which recognizes the muscular pressure waves, or (2) by an accelerometer that identifies the postural changes and the body movements related to physical activity. Both types of sensors are housed inside the pacemaker's case.

Unfortunately, these sensors respond to artifacts not related to body movements like laughing and coughing, but some of the relevant efforts, as isometric or slow but tiresome exercise, mental stress, and metabolic inadequacy, remain not registered. The possible mismatch between exercise intensity and the required heart rate increase represents the main limitations of activity sensors.

The sensors based on QT interval and minute ventilation (MV) provide pacing rates more closely and specifically related to physical and mental stress requirements [10].

Minute ventilation, the product of respiratory rate and tidal volume, is a physiological indicator that correlates well with metabolic demand [11]. This parameter, which also correlates linearly with heart rate, can be derived from variations in transthoracic and intracardiac impedance signals [12]. The voltage is measured as a response to the current injected between the proximal ventricular or atrial electrode and the pacemaker casing [13].

No single sensor can reproduce all the activities of daily life. Combining different sensors might more closely mimic intrinsic heart rate. For example, the combination of an activity sensor for getting a rapid response and a bioimpedance-based minute ventilation (MV) sensor, providing delayed but close to metabolic demand response, could be a solution [14].

4.2 Bioimpedance-based sensing

The most trustworthy sensing methods for the monitoring and control of pacing rate rely on measurement of electrical impedance, implementations of which are developed by Estonian scientists in collaboration with St. Jude Medical (USA/Sweden) during the period of 1999–2006. The variations of thorax impedance, measured between the tip of the pacing lead in the right ventricle and the case of pacemaker, give us lung impedance containing information about both the respiration rate and tidal volume. Using some soft computing method, e.g., fuzzy logic, we can evaluate the metabolic demand of the body and obtain a satisfactory pacing rate [15]. Implantable impedance measurement units were developed [16, 17]. Moreover, stroke volume and cardiac output are retrieved when measuring the impedance inside the right ventricle [18–20]. Finally, the balance condition between energy supply and consumption of myocardium has been calculated, and the maximal pacing rate was found to avoid over pacing [21]. Dangerously low pacing rate limit was also defined from the impedance measurements. A closed-loop control of the pacing rate by sensing of cardiac output has been discussed [22].

Both technology and clinical treatment methods have changed since the first cardiac devices developed during the twenty-first century. Diversity of cardiac pacing modes is available nowadays [23] for helping patients [24, 25]; some newest of these are considered in the next four chapters of the present book.

5. Novel indications and solutions presented in this book

Chapter 2 [26] presents the indications for cardiac devices, including pacemakers, cardiac resynchronization therapy (CRT) devices, and implantable cardioverter defibrillators (ICD). Contraindications due to different health conditions of patients are considered [24–27]. Pacemaker therapy is the treatment of bradycardia. An aging population increases the use of permanent pacemakers. Leadless pacing is a new landmark in the development of pacemaker technology but still limited to pacing in the right ventricle, only. The aim of CRT is to improve synchrony in the heart's contraction and avoid ventrical fibrillation (VF) by delivering a shock during the myocardial refractory period of cardiac cycle. The CRT devices are recommended for the treatment of atrial arrhythmias and ventricular tachycardia (VT). Around 30% of patients suffer from chronic heart failure (HF). Avoidance of sudden cardiac death (SCD) possibility in heart failure (HF) cases is also a task of CRT devices. The CRT with the ability to work as a cardiac defibrillator is termed as CRT-D, whereas the term CRT-P designates solely a pacing function. One major cause of death worldwide is sudden cardiac death SCD, which can be prevented most effectively by the aid of a specific device—the implantable cardiac defibrillator (ICD).

The subcutaneous ICD (S-ICD) is introduced in Chapter 3 [28]. This important advancement in defibrillation therapy obviates the need for a transvenous lead, the most frequent complication maker with transvenous devices. Unfortunately, the

S-ICD is appropriate for patients who require only rescue defibrillation. It cannot be used when the pacing against bradycardia or tachycardia is needed. Lead failure is the most frequent source of complication requiring surgical revision. Extraction of leads may cause devastating complications, including death.

Chapter 4 [29] deals with leadless or transcatheter pacemakers [30, 31] that have been introduced to the market some years ago with important benefits and some limitations. These devices are entirely implantable within the right ventricle. Thus, the transvenous pacing leads and pacemaker pockets are not needed anymore. This reduces the risk of infections and lead-related problems. Unfortunately, only the pacing in the right ventricle is available. Atrial sensing, anti-tachycardia pacing, and A/V synchrony are not possible, but the rate response by the aid of programmable accelerometer works.

Chapter 5 [32] explains that underdiagnosed atrial fibrillation (AF) may be potentially life-threatening arrhythmia, the appearance of which is episodic. Therefore, long-term day-and-night monitoring is required. Though the implantable cardiac monitors are in use for years already [25], the surgery is not reasonable in many cases. The chapter introduces a new user-friendly device that allows for frequent self-monitoring of the heart rhythm. This thumb ECG wearable device is a small format, patient-friendly device that can be used to monitor their heart rhythm regularly and continuously. Clinicians monitor the results by accessing a secure portal via an ordinary laptop computer. Bluetooth and mobile phone communication are available.

6. Summary

The present chapter reviews the developments of the implantable heart rhythm management from its dawn to mature technology. The book as a whole provides information about today's achievements in the field of cardiac pacing and monitoring with a view to the future.

Conflict of interest

The author has received financial and technical support in frames of the research agreements with St. Jude Medical and Guidant/Boston Scientific in 1999–2006.

Author details

Mart Min
Thomas Johann Seebeck Department of Electronics, Tallinn University of Technology, Tallinn, Estonia

*Address all correspondence to: mart.min@ttu.ee

References

[1] Aquilina O. A brief history of cardiac pacing. Images in Paediatric Cardiology. 2006;**8**(2):17-81

[2] Greatbatch W. US patent 3,057,356; Filed July 22, 1960

[3] Greatbatch W. US patent 3,723,183; Filed Feb 4, 1971

[4] Berkovits BV. US Patent 3,345,990; Filed Oct 19, 1964

[5] Berkovits BV. US Patent 3,595242; Filed Mar 26, 1969

[6] Gerber TC, Nishimura RA, Holmes DR, Lloyd MA, Zehr KJ, Tajik J, et al. Review: Left ventricular and biventricular pacing in congestive heart failure. Mayo Clinic Proceedings. 2001;**76**(8):803-812

[7] Corbisiero R, Muller D. Profile of St. Jude Medical's Allure Quadra quadripolar pacemaker system for cardiac resynchronization therapy. Expert Review of Medical Devices. 2014;**12**(1): 1-8. DOI: 10.1586/17434440.2015.984686

[8] Voukydis PC, Krasner JL. A physiologically regulated cardiac pacemaker. British Journal of Experimental Pathology. 1967;**48**(1):118-123

[9] Hayes DL, Furman S. Cardiac pacing: How it started, where we are, where we are going. Pacing and Clinical Electrophysiology. 2004;**27**(5):693-704

[10] Treese N et al. Ventilation and heart rate response during exercise in normals: Relevance for rate variable pacing. PACE. 1993;**16**:1693-1700

[11] Soucie LP et al. Correlation of the heart rate-minute ventilation relationship with clinical date: Relevance to rate-adaptive pacing. PACE. 1997;**20**:1913-1918

[12] Vai F, Bonnet JL, Ritter P, Pioger G. Relationship between heart rate and minute ventilation, tidal volume and respiratory rate during brief and low level exercise. PACE. 1988;**11**:1860-1865

[13] Nappholtz T, Valenta H, Maloney J, Simmons T. Electrode configurations for a respiratory impedance measurement suitable for rate responsive pacing. PACE. 1986;**9**:960-964

[14] Dell'Orto S, Valli P, Greco EM. Minute ventilation sensors can change the heart rate according to variations of respiratory rate and tidal volume. In: Sensors for rate responsive pacing. Indian Pacing and Electrophysiology Journal. 2004;**4**(3):137-145

[15] Min M, Parve T, Kink A. Thoracic bioimpedance as a basis for pacing control. Annals of the New York Academy of Sciences. 1999;**873**(1):155-166

[16] Min M, Parve T, Kukk V, Kuhlberg A. An implantable analyzer of bio-impedance dynamics: Mixed signal approach. IEEE Transactions on Instrumentation and Measurement. 2002;**51**(4):674-678

[17] Min M, Parve T. Improvement of lock-in electrical bio-impedance analyzer for implantable medical devices. IEEE Transactions on Instrumentaion and Measurement. 2002;**56**(3):968-974

[18] Min M, Kink A, Parve T. Rate adaptive pacemaker. US Patent 6,885,892; 2005

[19] Min M, Kink A, Parve T. Rate adaptive pacemaker using impedance measurements and stroke volume calculations. US Patent 6,975,903; 2005

[20] Kink A, Min M, Parve T, Rätsep I. Device and method for monitoring

cardiac pacing rate. US Patent 7,894,900; 2011

[21] Min M, Kink A, Parve T, Rätsep I. Bioimpedance based control of rate limits in artificial cardiac pacing. In: Proc. BioMED2005 Conference; Innsbruck (Austria). Canada: ACTA Press; 2005. pp. 697-703

[22] Kink A, Salo RW, Min M, Parve T, Rätsep I. Intracardiac electrical bioimpedance as a basis for controlling of pacing rate limits. In: Proc. of the 28th IEEE EMBS Annual International Conference; 30 Aug–3 Sept 2006; New York City (USA): IEEE; 2006. pp. 6308-6311

[23] Erol-Yilmaz A. Studies on cardiac pacing: Emphasis on pacemaker sensors and cardiac resynchronization therapy [thesis]. Amsterdam (Netherlands): Amsterdam University; 2006

[24] Hauser RG. Heart Stories: About Patients and the Great Pioneers who Saved Them. Florida, USA; 2016

[25] Giada F, Bertaglia E, Reimers B, Noventa D, Raviele A. Current and emerging indications for implantable cardiac monitors. Pacing and Clinical Electrophysiology. 2012;**35**(9):1169-1178

[26] Åberg I, Mattsson G, Magnusson P. Clinical indications for therapeutic cardiac devices. Chapter 2. In: Min M, editor. Cardiac Pacing and Monitoring: New Methods, Modern Devices. London: IntechOpen; 2019

[27] Hayes DL. Permanent cardiac pacing: Overview of devices and indications. UpToDate [Internet]. 2019. Available from: https://www.uptodate.com/contents/permanent-cardiac-pacing-overview-of-devices-and-indications [Accessed: 2019-03-15]

[28] Magnusson P, Pergolizzi JV, LeQuang JA. The Subcutaneous implantable cardioverter-defibrillator. Chapter 3. In: Min M, editor. Cardiac Pacing and Monitoring: New Methods, Modern Devices. London: IntechOpen; 2019

[29] Magnusson P, Pergolizzi JV, LeQuang JA. Leadless pacemakers. Chapter 4. In: Min M, editor. Cardiac Pacing and Monitoring: New Methods, Modern Devices. London: IntechOpen; 2019

[30] Tjong FV, Reddy VY. Permanent leadless cardiac pacemaker therapy: A comprehensive review. Circulation. 2017;**135**(15):1458-1470

[31] Della Rocca DG, Gianni C, Di Biase L, Natale A, Amin Al-Ahmad A. Leadless pacemakers: State of the art and future perspectives. Cardiac Electrophysiology Clinics. 2018;**10**(1):17-29

[32] Magnusson P, Samuelsson M, Pergolizzi JV, Annabi H, LeQuang JA. Atrial fibrillation and the role of thumb ECGs. Ch. 5. In: Min M, editor. Cardiac Pacing and Monitoring: New Methods, Modern Devices. London: IntechOpen; 2019

Chapter 2

Clinical Indications for Therapeutic Cardiac Devices

Ida Åberg, Gustav Mattsson and Peter Magnusson

Abstract

Both technology and clinical indications have changed since the first cardiac devices. Choosing the right therapy, or abstaining from it, is the key to good clinical management. Pacemakers effectively reduce symptoms of bradycardia, prevent syncope in patients with sick sinus syndrome, and reduce mortality in high-degree atrioventricular block. Cardiac resynchronization therapy improves symptoms and survival in heart failure patients with reduced ejection fraction and ventricular dyssynchrony. Implantable cardioverter defibrillators terminate life-threatening ventricular arrhythmias and are indicated for the prevention of sudden cardiac death, either as secondary prevention in survivors of ventricular fibrillation or ventricular tachycardia with hemodynamic compromise or as primary prevention due to heart failure with reduced ejection fraction or other miscellaneous diseases. More recently, leadless pacemakers and subcutaneous implantable cardioverter defibrillators have been developed as alternatives in specific conditions.

Keywords: bradycardia, cardiac devices, cardiac resynchronization therapy, heart failure, implantable cardioverter defibrillator, indication, pacemaker, sudden cardiac death

1. Introduction

"Those who suffer from frequent and strong faints without any manifest cause die suddenly", Hippocrates stated more than 2000 years ago [1]. This is likely a description of arrhythmia-related death, which nowadays often is avoidable due to the improvements in diagnostics and treatment the world has seen since antiquity.

The majority of patients receiving a pacemaker today are above the age of 65, owing to increasing problems with impulse generation and conduction with age [2]. With the world population getting older, the prevalence of permanent pacemakers will likely continue to rise [3]. This chapter aims to present a concise description of current guidelines regarding the indications for cardiac devices, including pacemakers, cardiac resynchronization therapy (CRT), and implantable cardioverter defibrillators (ICD) (**Figure 1**).

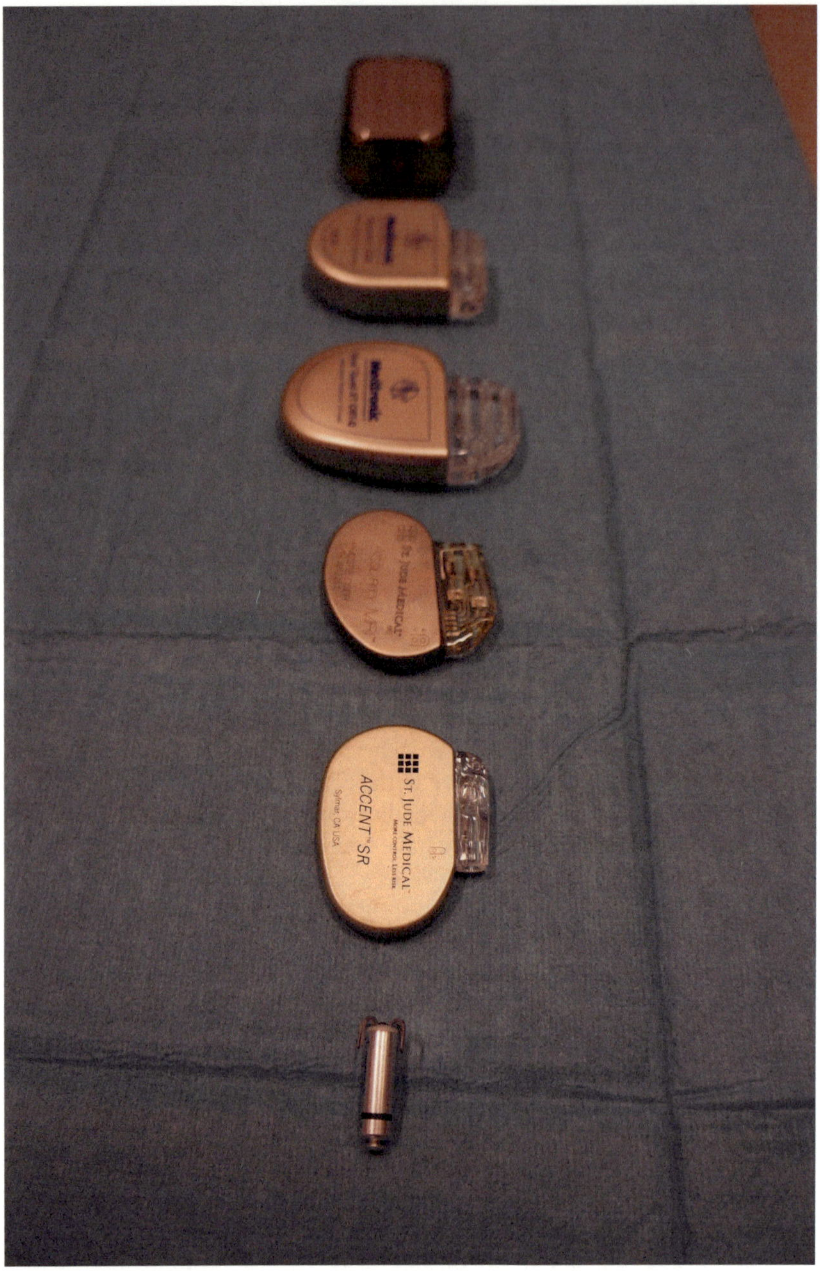

Figure 1.
Cardiac devices. From the top: older pacemaker, dual-chamber implantable cardioverter defibrillator, cardiac resynchronization therapy-defibrillator, dual-chamber pacemaker, single-chamber pacemaker, and leadless pacemaker.

2. Pacemaker therapy

The medical properties of electricity have been known for some time. The physicians of ancient Rome treated acute gout with electric sea creatures. Alexander von Humboldt tested the theory of electrical conduction in biological tissue on himself. The first artificial pacemaker, powered by a hand-cranked motor, was invented by Albert Hyman in 1932. The first patient to receive an implantable pacemaker, Arne Larsson, had to wait until 1958, when he underwent the procedure at the Karolinska

University Hospital in Stockholm. He outlived both the surgeon Åke Senning and the engineer Rune Elmqvist who developed the system [1].

2.1 Etiology

The most common etiology of bradycardia leading to pacemaker implantation is conduction tissue fibrosis, but there are several others etiologies responsible for slow heart rates according to data from registers, for example the Swedish pacemaker registry [4]. Some of these are reversible, such as infection/inflammation, metabolic conditions, and medications while others are congenital such as third-degree atrioventricular (AV) block associated with maternal systemic lupus erythematosus [5].

2.2 Pacing mode

A code of four to five letters is used to describe the pacing mode. The first letter indicates where pacing occurs (where A stands for atrium, V for ventricle, and D for dual); the second describes which chamber is sensed. In the third position, the letters I (inhibit), T (trigger), or D (dual) are used to describe in which way the device responds to sensed events. An R in the fourth position means that rate response (increased pacing rate during physical exertion) is active. Finally, a fifth letter is occasionally used to describe where multicenter pacing is employed (A, V, or D) [6].

2.3 Rate response

The purpose of rate response is to increase the heart rate in response to altered demand, and there are different solutions available to achieve this. Activity sensors are widely used; one example is the accelerometer that identifies postural changes and movement. Minute ventilation sensors can change the heart rate according to variations of respiratory rate and tidal volume [7].

2.4 Pacemaker syndrome

The pacemaker syndrome is a condition brought on by the loss of AV synchrony caused by ventricular pacing. There are no specific diagnostic criteria, but symptoms include orthopnea, dyspnea upon exertion, orthostatic hypotension, and syncope. The mode selection trial (MOST), a prospective study of patients with sick sinus syndrome (SSS) randomized to VVIR or DDDR pacing, concluded that the incidence of pacemaker syndrome was 19.7% at 4 years after implantation. The incidence of pacemaker syndrome varies between less than 2 and 83% in multiple studies [8].

2.5 Mode switch

This is crucial in patients with paroxysmal atrial tachyarrhythmias. The cut-off for mode-switch is based on sensing of electrical activity of an atrial lead and is programmable, typically 180 beats per minute. Atrial flutter activity is sometimes hidden in the so-called post-ventricular blanking period and often requires reprogramming. Furthermore, nonphysiological electrical activity may lead to oversensing which results in mode-switch.

2.6 Indications for permanent pacing

In bradycardia caused by reversible etiologies, permanent pacing is not warranted, and temporary pacing should instead be considered. Generally, once reversible causes for bradycardia are excluded, the indication for pacing is based on the severity of bradycardia rather than its etiology [9]. It should be noted though that symptomatic sinus bradycardia as a result of medical therapy is an indication for permanent pacing if there are no alternative treatment options [10].

2.6.1 Sinus node dysfunction

Persistent sinus bradycardia, chronotropic incompetence, and sinus arrest can all be seen in sinus node disease (SND), a condition that primarily affects the elderly [10]. When diagnosing chronotropic incompetence (the inability to increase the heart rate as a response to activity or other demands), the fact that heart rate is affected by aging, medication, and physical conditioning must be taken into account. Exercise testing is the basis for diagnosis [11]. It is important to separate physiological bradycardia from inappropriate bradycardia, since sinus bradycardia in trained athletes is normal and not an indication for pacemaker therapy [10].

2.6.1.1 Persistent bradycardia

In patients with SND, pacing has not been proven to prolong survival and is therefore used to relieve symptoms. Symptoms of bradycardia include impaired tolerance to exercise, symptoms of heart failure (HF), syncope, and more subtle symptoms like dizziness and forgetfulness. Untreated patients with SSS, however, are commonly affected by systemic thromboembolism [9]. A significant reduction in stroke and atrial fibrillation (AF) among these patients has been seen with AAI or DDD compared with VVI. The DANPACE trial shows that the incidence of paroxysmal AF is higher with AAIR pacing than DDDR, and there is a two-fold increase in the risk of re-operation [12]. In the Canadian Trial of Physiologic Pacing (CTOPP) where physiologic pacing (dual-chamber or atrial) was compared to ventricular pacing in patients with symptomatic bradycardia, a reduction in the risk of AF was seen for patients who received dual-chamber pacing. No significant reduction in the risk of stroke, death, or hospitalization for HF in the first 3 years after implantation was seen with dual-chamber pacing, but the risk of perioperative complications was significantly higher in this group [13]. The MOST trial compared ventricular- to dual-chamber pacing in patients with SSS, and no reduction in stroke with dual-chamber pacing was observed. However, a reduction of AF, signs and symptoms of HF, and a slight improvement in quality of life was seen [14]. Between 0.6 and 1.9% of all patients with SND develop AV block every year, which can of course be a problem when AAIR is used [9]. Rate response should be considered (class IIa recommendation) in people with SND and chronotropic incompetence according to the guidelines of the European Society of Cardiology (ESC). The indication is strengthened in those who are young and physically active. There is evidence for improvement in quality of life and exercise capacity with VVIR compared to VVI. When it comes to comparing DDD with DDDR there have been inconsistent results [9]. In extrinsic (functional, induced by for example drugs or high vagal tone) bradycardia, the prognosis is benign, and pacing is only indicated to prevent recurrent syncope [9].

2.6.1.2 Intermittent bradycardia

Documented symptomatic bradycardia due to sinoatrial block or sinus arrest in patients with intrinsic SND (including the brady-tachy form) is a class I recommendation for pacemaker therapy by the ESC [9]. When there is no documented correlation between symptoms and electrocardiography (ECG), people with intrinsic sinus node dysfunction may still be candidates for cardiac pacing if they have experienced syncope and there are documented asymptomatic ventricular pauses of more than 3 seconds. This does not apply to young, well-trained, or medicated persons and during sleep. Alternative explanations such as hypotension should be ruled out before deciding on pacemaker therapy [9]. The recommendations regarding pacing mode for permanent bradycardia apply for intermittent bradycardia as well, based on the fact that there are not enough studies including only patients with intermittent bradycardia. Dual-chamber pacing is preferred to reduce the risk of pacemaker syndrome [9].

2.6.2 Atrioventricular block

2.6.2.1 Persistent bradycardia

Pacing improves survival in people with AV block (third-degree and second-degree type 2), as well as prevents recurrence of syncope. There are no randomized controlled trials (RCTs), but observational studies from the beginning of the pacemaker era suggest this. One study describes a one-year mortality of about 50% in patients with complete AV block [15]. Therefore, pacemaker therapy is recommended by the ESC in these patients, even if they are asymptomatic [9]. Permanent pacing is controversial in second-degree type 1 AV block; although not if it is symptomatic or the conduction delay is situated at intra- or infra-His levels, in these cases pacing should be considered (class of recommendation IIa). If the QRS complex is wide, development of complete AV block is more likely [9].

Studies have shown that above one quarter of people with VVI develop pacemaker syndrome. Dual-chamber pacing reduces the risk of these symptoms. Since they require an additional lead and have longer implantation times and a higher risk of complications, dual-chamber devices are more expensive. When the risk of AF and pacemaker syndrome is taken into account, the cost difference is small over a five-year period. Since there is no reduction in morbidity or mortality with dual-chamber pacing compared to ventricular pacing, the choice should be made on an individual basis where increased risk of complications and cost is considered [9]. The United Kingdom Pacing and Cardiovascular Events (UKPACE) trial compared dual-chamber pacing to ventricular pacing in elderly patients with high grade AV block and found that pacing mode does not affect survival, and in contrast with the CTOPP trial, no reduction in AF in dual-chamber compared to ventricular pacing was seen. Fixed-rate single-chamber pacing was associated with an increased risk of stroke, transient ischemic attack, and thromboembolism compared with dual-chamber pacing, but there was no difference between the rate-adaptive single-chamber and dual-chamber groups [16].

In permanent AF and AV block, the ESC recommendation (class I recommendation) is ventricular pacing with rate response [9].

2.6.2.2 Intermittent bradycardia

Correlations between symptoms and ECG are not as important in intrinsic third- or second-degree AV block as it is in SSS. The ESC states that cardiac pacing is indicated in people suffering from intrinsic intermittent AV block, regardless of documentation of correlation between symptoms and ECG findings [9].

2.6.3 Suspected (undocumented) bradycardia

In patients with syncope, the presence of bundle branch block (BBB) suggests that the cause may be complete heart block. In spite of this, less than half of patients with

BBB and syncope are diagnosed with cardiac syncope. According to the ISSUE 1 study and the Bradycardia detection in Bundle Branch Block (B4) study [17] (that included patients with normal or preserved systolic function), it is safe to wait until the correct diagnosis is made before starting cardiac pacing [9]. ICD or CRT-D should be considered in patients with syncope who have BBB and HF, previous myocardial infarction, or ejection fraction (EF) ≤ 35%. This is because a high incidence of total and sudden cardiac death (SCD) has been observed in patients with BBB, and mostly those with HF, previous myocardial infarction, or low EF [9]. In patients with BBB who have experienced syncope but have normal EF, an electrophysiological study should be considered. If this study is abnormal, pacing is a class I recommendation in the ESC guidelines [9]. If the electrophysiological study is normal, an insertable cardiac monitor should be considered since EPS cannot rule out intermittent or paroxysmal AV block [9].

Cardiac pacing is generally indicated in alternating BBB (block involving all three fascicles on successive ECGs) since it is known to progress toward AV block fast, even if there is no history of syncope [9]. Asymptomatic BBB is not an indication for pacemaker therapy. In some cases though, patients with unexplained syncope and BBB are candidates for pacemaker therapy, especially old people with unpredictable syncope [9].

2.6.4 Carotid sinus syncope

Carotid sinus syncope is defined as a drop in blood pressure of 50 mmHg or asystole of more than 3 s as a result of carotid sinus massage [9]. Dual-chamber pacing is indicated when asystole of 6 s and syncope follows carotid sinus massage (to be performed for a full 10 s, supine and erect), and the patient has recurrent and unpredictable syncope [9].

2.6.5 Tilt-induced vasovagal syncope

Tilt-induced vasovagal syncope often affects young people and is in itself a benign condition. When deciding whether to implant a pacemaker, this must be taken into consideration [9]. Pacing may be considered (class IIb recommendation according to ESC) in these patients if they suffer from recurrent and unpredictable episodes, are older than 40 years, and have a documented cardio-inhibitory reflex, but only after other therapies have failed [9]. As with carotid sinus syncope, dual-chamber pacing is recommended [9].

2.7 Indications for pacing in specific conditions

2.7.1 Pacing in acute myocardial infarction

Primary angioplasty and thrombolytic therapy have led to a decrease in AV block associated with acute myocardial infarction, but it still occurs and when it does, mortality is high [10]. When advanced second- or third-degree AV block is seen with left bundle branch block (LBBB) or when right bundle branch block occurs with left anterior or posterior fascicular block, the prognosis is particularly bad [10]. Intraventricular conduction delays develop as a result of extensive damage to the myocardium, meaning greater injury to the heart than an isolated electrical problem [10]. If the AV block is expected to be temporary, permanent pacemaker therapy should be avoided [10]. AV block associated with acute myocardial infarction resolves spontaneously in 2–7 days in most cases [9]. Permanent AV pacing is recommended by the American Heart Association (AHA) in persistent and symptomatic second- or third-degree AV block following acute myocardial infarction. Persistent second-degree AV block in the His-Purkinje system associated with alternating bundle branch block also constitutes an indication for permanent ventricular pacing, as well as third-degree AV block within or below the His-Purkinje system following ST elevation myocardial infarction. In the case of associated bundle branch block, permanent ventricular pacing is indicated in transient advanced second-degree and third-degree infra-nodal AV block according to AHA, whereas ESC states that there is no evidence that pacing improves outcomes in these patients [9, 10]. Permanent AV pacing may be considered in the case of persistent second-degree or third-degree AV block at the AV node level, even if there are no symptoms, according to the AHA [10]. According to the ESC, the recommendations for pacemaker therapy in permanent AV block following acute myocardial infarction are the same as those for AV block of other etiologies [9].

2.7.2 Pacing after cardiac surgery, transcatheter aortic valve implantation, and heart transplantation

Both AV block and SND may appear as complications after cardiac interventions, and if they persist, permanent pacing must be considered. An observation time of up to 7 days is recommended before implanting a permanent pacemaker in high degree or complete AV block following cardiac surgery or transcatheter aortic valve implantation. A shorter observation time can be used in case of complete AV block with a low escape rhythm, where resolution is not likely. SND as a result of cardiac surgery or heart transplantation should be observed from 5 days up to some weeks before deciding on pacemaker therapy [9].

2.7.3 Pacing in children and in congenital heart disease

When implanting a pacemaker in a young person, several considerations have to be made. For one, they will have the pacemaker for a whole lifetime, increasing the risk of experiencing complications sometime during this period. They usually have higher activity levels than adults, and because of this and the fact that they grow the risk of stress on the device and electrode dislodgement is increased. The presence of right to left-shunt is a contraindication for endocardial leads; hence, epicardial pacing is used instead in this congenital defect. Small body size and the absence of transvenous access are other reasons why epicardial pacing is often preferred in children. Second-degree type 2 and third-degree AV block are indications (class I according to ESC) for pacemaker therapy in children who are symptomatic or if any of the following risk factors are present: ventricular dysfunction, prolonged QTc interval, complex ventricular ectopy, wide QRS complex escape rhythm, slow ventricular rate (<50 beats per minute, ventricular pauses more than three times the cycle length of the underlying rhythm) with or without symptoms. For children without any risk factors, the ESC states that pacing may be considered in high-degree and complete AV block, adding that opinions regarding the benefit of pacing differ. Pacemaker therapy is indicated for children with SND if they are symptomatic and there is a clear correlation between symptoms and bradycardia. The decision to implant a pacemaker in a child should be made after discussion with pediatric cardiologists, and it is recommended that it is done in a specialized center [9].

2.7.4 Pacing in hypertrophic cardiomyopathy

Patients who have symptoms because of left ventricular outflow tract obstruction can be treated medically, surgically, with septal alcohol ablation, and sequential AV pacing [9]. Sequential AV pacing is an alternative when myectomy or septal alcohol ablation are contraindicated or when the risk of AV block after these procedures is considered high [9].

2.7.5 Pacing in pregnancy

Complete heart block with a slow escape rhythm with wide QRS complexes should be treated with pacemaker implantation during pregnancy, using echo-guidance or electro-anatomic navigation to avoid fluoroscopy. The procedure is safe, especially when the fetus is beyond 8 weeks of gestation. In case of stable, junctional escape rhythm with narrow complexes, pacemaker implantation can be delayed until after delivery [9].

2.7.6 Leadless pacemakers

Malfunction of the electrodes is the most common cause of surgical pacemaker revision. Pocket hematoma and erosion are other complications associated with pacemaker implantation [18]. There are currently two self-contained leadless pacemaker systems available: Nanostim™ and Micra™. Nanostim™ has been evaluated in the prospective nonrandomized study LEADLESS, and the complication-free rate compares favorably with traditional pacemaker systems [18]. As for Micra™, the risk of major complications in the first 12 months after implantation was 48% lower compared to historical control patients with transvenous systems [19]. Currently, solely the VVI-mode is available via leadless pacemaker systems. Considering this, the higher cost and the fact that there is not much experience outside clinical trials with these systems yet, use of leadless pacemakers should for now be reserved for when VVI-mode is indicated and transvenous leads are unfeasible or undesirable.

2.8 Emergency temporary pacing

Bradycardia can be a life-threatening condition where immediate action is crucial. When the hemodynamics is affected resulting in symptoms of acute HF, ischemic chest pain, or signs of shock, the first step is to administer atropine intravenously. If atropine is not effective or appropriate, a continuous infusion with beta-adrenergic agonists such as isoproterenol, dopamine, or epinephrine is sometimes needed to uphold an adequate pulse until pacemaker therapy can be initiated. Another alternative is transcutaneous pacing, which can be used while waiting for implantation of a temporary transvenous- or permanent pacemaker [20]. The pads are preferably attached with anterior-posterior placement and are then connected to the defibrillator/monitor [21]. Transcutaneous pacing can be performed on a conscious patient, but sedation is preferred [21, 22]. During transcutaneous pacing, the patient must be monitored closely with ECG and with regard to hemodynamic stability [9]. Seeing that there are a number of risks associated with temporary transvenous pacing (for example, accidental extraction of the pacemaker lead by the patient, risk of infection, and thromboembolic events), the ESC recommends avoiding this treatment if possible, and otherwise keeping the treatment time as brief as possible [9].

3. The implantable cardioverter defibrillator

The first patient to receive an ICD was a woman who had survived repeated episodes of ventricular fibrillation (VF) and continued to experience arrhythmias refractory to medical therapy [23]. This was at The Johns Hopkins Hospital in the US in 1980, after extensive work by Michel Mirowski and his colleagues. After the death of his mentor, who suffered from recurrent ventricular tachyarrhythmias, Mirowski's goal was to create a device that could monitor the heart rhythm and administer a defibrillating shock to treat life-threatening tachyarrhythmias [24]. Today the ICD is the treatment of choice for both primary and secondary prevention of SCD due to VT/VF [25].

3.1 Etiology

Every year, cardiovascular diseases cause around 17 million deaths worldwide, of which SCD makes up approximately 25% [25]. The vast majority of these deaths are due to ventricular tachyarrhythmias. According to epidemiological data, 80% of the fatal arrhythmias occur as a consequence of structural coronary artery abnormalities. Dilated- and hypertrophic cardiomyopathies are the second most common reasons for SCD [26]. Among the young, channelopathies, cardiomyopathies, myocarditis, and drug-induced arrhythmias are more common, while coronary artery disease, valvular heart diseases, and HF predominate in older individuals [25].

3.2 Cardioversion and antitachycardia pacing

Cardioversion implies that shock delivery is synchronized with the QRS complex to avoid inducing VF by delivering a shock during the refractory period of the cardiac cycle, and it is recommended for the treatment of several supraventricular arrhythmias and monomorphic ventricular tachycardia (VT) with pulses. It should not be used to treat VF or pulseless or polymorphic VT, since these arrhythmias require unsynchronized high-energy doses, also known as defibrillation [27]. Antitachycardia pacing is an alternative way to terminate monomorphic ventricular arrhythmias; it can reduce the number of shocks and is generally tolerated well since it is rarely noticed by the patient. The mechanism is that a short sequence of pacemaker pulses (typically 8–12), with a rate slightly faster than the detected tachycardia, is delivered as a response to ventricular arrhythmia. The success rate varies but has in some cohorts been shown to exceed 90% [28].

3.3 Indications for ICD

In patients with high risk of SCD, ICD therapy prevents SCD and prolongs life (given that life expectancy is not for other reasons less than 1–2 years) [25]. Both patients who have experienced previous ventricular arrhythmias and those who are at increased risk of future arrhythmia can be protected by ICD therapy.

3.3.1 Secondary prevention

In patients who have survived an episode of documented VF or VT that is not hemodynamically tolerated, ICD is a class I recommendation according to the ESC, provided that there are no reversible causes and that the expected survival with good functional status is at least 1 year [25]. Recurrent sustained VT (not including the first 48 hours after myocardial infarction) in patients who are treated with optimal medical therapy and have a normal left ventricular EF (LVEF) should be considered for ICD therapy (class IIa recommendation). Survival must be expected for at least a year with good functional status [25]. Three trials have studied the effect of ICD compared to medical treatment as secondary prevention in patients who have survived VF or sustained VT: the antiarrhythmics vs.

implantable defibrillator (AVID) study (patients with VT had syncope or serious cardiac symptoms and an LVEF of 40% or less) [29], the Cardiac Arrest Study Hamburg (CASH) (patients were survivors of cardiac arrest secondary to documented ventricular arrhythmias) [30], and the Canadian Implantable Defibrillator Study (CIDS) (patients with VT had syncope or cardiac symptoms and an LVEF of 35% or less; patients with unmonitored syncope and subsequent documentation of VT were also included) [31]. The AVID study showed an increase in overall survival in the ICD group. In the CASH study, the reduction in all-cause mortality in the ICD group did not reach statistical significance but there was a 61% reduction in SCD. The reduction in all-cause mortality and SCD seen in the ICD group in the CIDS study was not statistically significant. A meta-analysis of these three trials concluded that there is a 28% reduction in total mortality with ICD therapy compared to amiodarone, mainly due to a 50% reduction in arrhythmic mortality [32]. In the following sections, current guidelines regarding secondary prevention in specific circumstances are addressed.

3.3.1.1 Acute coronary syndromes

Approximately 6% of patients with acute coronary syndrome experience VT/VF within 48 hours after the first symptoms, the majority during or before reperfusion therapy [25, 33]. As stated above, ICD is recommended after an episode of VF or hemodynamically compromising VT, unless the episode occurred within 48 hours of myocardial infarction, in a patient who receives optimal medical treatment [25].

3.3.1.2 Cardiomyopathies

In patients with hypertrophic cardiomyopathy, dilated cardiomyopathy, left ventricular noncompaction cardiomyopathy, and arrhythmogenic right ventricular cardiomyopathy, ICD therapy is indicated after a survived episode of cardiac arrest due to VT/VF, or in patients who have experienced syncope or hemodynamic compromise because of spontaneous sustained VT—in accordance with the guidelines in general [25]. When it comes to arrhythmogenic right ventricular cardiomyopathy, the ESC suggests that ICD should be considered (class IIa) in patients who have experienced hemodynamically well tolerated sustained VT as well. For patients with light-chain amyloidosis or hereditary transthyretin-associated amyloidosis who have had a sustained VT with hemodynamic impact, and have a life expectancy of more than a year with good functional status, ICD should be considered. This recommendation is upgraded to a class I (is recommended) regarding restrictive cardiomyopathy [25].

3.3.1.3 Hereditary primary arrhythmia syndromes

ICD therapy and beta-blockers are recommended for patients with long QT syndrome and previous cardiac arrest and should be considered in these patients if they have experienced syncope or VT while on an adequate dose of beta-blockers [25]. In catecholaminergic polymorphic VT, ICD as an addition to beta-blockers is recommended after a survived cardiac arrest, recurrent syncope, or polymorphic/bidirectional VT during treatment with optimal medical therapy [25]. In short QT syndrome and Brugada syndrome, ICD is recommended for patients who have survived a cardiac arrest or those who have experienced documented spontaneous sustained VT [25]. In Brugada syndrome, an ICD may be indicated in primary prevention, especially when syncope is likely due to an arrhythmic event [34].

3.3.2 Primary prevention

3.3.2.1 Heart failure

In the Sudden Cardiac Death in Heart Failure (SCD-HeFT) trial a decrease in the overall mortality of 23% was seen in patients with both ischemic and nonischemic HF in New York Heart Association (NYHA) functional class II and III and an LVEF of 35% or less who received an ICD [35]. An LVEF of 35% or less and symptomatic HF (NYHA II-III) after 3 months of optimal medication is a class I indication for ICD therapy according to the ESC (provided that the expected survival with good functional status is at least 1 year) [25]. More recently, the DANISH trial randomized patients with symptomatic HF (LVEF of 35% or less) of nonischemic origin to ICD therapy or usual clinical care, and found no overall survival benefit with ICD therapy, although the risk of SCD was halved [36]. However, all-cause mortality was significantly reduced by ICD in patients younger than 59 years old. There is currently no indication for ICD therapy in patients with HF in NYHA class IV, unless they are listed for heart transplantation since their risk of SCD is generally high and the wait is often a year or more [25].

3.3.2.2 Acute coronary syndromes

In 1996, results from the MADIT trial were published, showing that in patients with a prior myocardial infarction, NYHA class I-III, LVEF of less than 35%, a documented asymptomatic nonsustained VT, and nonsuppressible VT on an electrophysiological study, prophylactic ICD therapy leads to improved survival [37]. The MADIT-II trial enrolled patients with reduced left ventricular function (LVEF 30% or less) after myocardial infarction and found that the patients who received ICD therapy had a 31% decrease in all-cause mortality [38]. LVEF should be assessed before discharge from the hospital in all patients with acute coronary syndrome, and re-assessed 6–12 weeks later, to evaluate whether or not primary prevention ICD implantation is indicated. As in nonischemic etiology with LVEF of 35% or lower, symptomatic HF (NYHA class II-III), expected survival with good functional status for at least 1 year, and optimal medical therapy for at least 3 months, ICD therapy is recommended (class I recommendation) by the ESC. At least 6 weeks must have passed since the myocardial infarction before deciding on ICD therapy [25]. The use of an ICD as prophylaxis in patients with a recent myocardial infarction (6–40 days previously) does not reduce the overall mortality; a reduction in SCD was offset by an increase in nonarrhythmic death [39]. Hence, ICD implantation within 40 days of acute myocardial infarction as primary prevention of SCD is generally not indicated but it may be considered in specific cases: preexisting impairment in LVEF, incomplete revascularization, and arrhythmia that occurs more than 48 hours after acute myocardial infarction [25].

3.3.2.3 Cardiomyopathies

The DEFINITE trial studied patients with nonischemic dilated cardiomyopathy with an EF of less than 36% and premature ventricular complexes or nonsustained VT, and found that ICD implantation significantly reduced the risk of SCD [40]. The same indications for ICD therapy regarding patients with symptomatic heart failure apply to patients with dilated cardiomyopathy and left ventricular noncompaction cardiomyopathy. In addition to this, ICD should be considered in patients with dilated cardiomyopathy who have a verified disease-causing LMNA mutation (frequently seen in patients with conduction diseases) and clinical risk factors [25].

Regarding primary prevention in HCM, a calculator that estimates the 5-year risk of SCD (HCM Risk-SCD) is recommended by the ESC to evaluate the need for ICD therapy in patients aged 16 or older. Based on the risk score, the class of recommendation regarding ICD therapy varies [25]. When it comes to primary prophylactic ICD in patients with arrhythmogenic right ventricular cardiomyopathy, the ESC suggests that ICD should be considered in patients who have experienced unexplained syncope. ICD may be considered in patients with arrhythmogenic right ventricular cardiomyopathy who have at least one risk factor for ventricular arrhythmias, including family history of premature SCD and extensive right ventricular disease. The risks of ICD therapy should be taken into account when considering it as primary prophylactic therapy [25]. Finally, ICD therapy should be considered in patients with Chagas disease (a cardiomyopathy caused by the parasite Trypanosoma cruzi) who have an EF of less than 40% [25].

3.3.2.4 Hereditary primary arrhythmia syndromes

In patients with long QT syndrome, ICD may be considered (as a complement to beta-blockers) in patients who are asymptomatic carriers of a pathogenic *KCNH2*- or *SCN5A*-mutation (high-risk genetic profiles) and have a QTc of more than 500 ms [25]. An ICD may be considered as primary prevention in short QT syndrome, if there is a family history of SCD and evidence of shortened QT in some of these patients. The available data is too scarce for any specific recommendations to be made regarding this. As for Brugada syndrome, primary prevention with an ICD should be considered in patients with a spontaneous type I ECG pattern and suspected arrhythmic syncope in their medical history, and may be considered in patients who develop VF during programmed ventricular stimulation [25].

3.3.2.5 Pediatric patients

A number of different etiologies are responsible for the risk of SCD in children: channelopathies, cardiomyopathies, and congenital heart disease. The same guidelines for when ICD is indicated apply to both adults and children, with the exception of dilated cardiomyopathy and advanced dysfunction of the left ventricle since the incidence of SCD is low in this group [25].

3.4 The subcutaneous ICD

This system is placed completely outside the thoracic cavity, eliminating problems with vascular access and transvenous leads. Subcutaneous ICD therapy is not appropriate for patients with bradycardia that requires pacing, for those who have indications for CRT or for those who need antitachycardia pacing. When these patients are excluded, subcutaneous defibrillators should be considered as an alternative to transvenous defibrillators (class IIa recommendation) in patients with an ICD indication [25]. According to the ESC, subcutaneous ICD could be considered (class IIb recommendation) as an alternative to transvenous defibrillators when there are difficulties with venous access, after ICD removal secondary to infection or in young patients who will require long-term ICD therapy [25].

3.5 The wearable cardioverter defibrillator

As the name suggests, this defibrillator is entirely external; defibrillator, leads and electrode pads are attached to a wearable vest. It may be considered for adult patients with reduced LVEF who are waiting for a more permanent solution (cardiac transplantation, transvenous implant) or those who are at a temporary risk of SCD, as in peripartum cardiomyopathy or active myocarditis [25, 41].

3.6 Contraindications and considerations

All through the European guidelines concerning ICD indications, it is emphasized that the expected survival with good functional status should be at least 1 year for ICD to be an option. As mentioned before, symptomatic HF with NYHA class IV is considered a contraindication, unless the patient is waiting for heart transplantation. VT or VF due to reversible causes should not be treated with ICD [25]. Psychiatric illness that might be aggravated due to ICD implantation is sometimes considered a contraindication [42], although it is not mentioned as such in the ESC guidelines. Up to a fifth of terminally ill patients with an ICD experience shocks in the last weeks of life, and deactivation of the ICD should be considered when the patient's condition worsens. This issue should be discussed before implantation and as the illness progresses [25]. A magnet placed over the ICD will deactivate tachyarrhythmia therapies, and this stops inappropriate defibrillations or unnecessary defibrillations at the end of life.

3.7 Health-related quality of life

In its guidelines, the ESC emphasizes the importance of discussing health-related quality of life issues with the patient before ICD implantation and during progression of the disease, by making it a class I recommendation. In addition to this, they recommend that patients who experience inappropriate shocks are assessed psychologically and treated for any distress [25]. Depression and anxiety are common in ICD patients; one systematic review reports anxiety in 8–63% of these patients and depression in 5–41% [43]. Similar effects on quality of life have been seen in patients with ICD and with medical therapy, with impairment in quality of life associated with adverse symptoms in both groups and experience of sporadic shocks in the ICD group [44]. Some patients develop post-traumatic stress disorder, and these symptoms have been associated with nonconstructive support (information that leads to insecurity and fear) from healthcare professionals; further studies are needed [45].

4. Cardiac resynchronization therapy

In around 30% of patients suffering from chronic HF, the conduction pathways are affected, leading to cardiac dyssynchrony [46]. The aim of CRT is to, as the name suggests, improve synchrony in the heart's contraction [9]. Patients eligible for this therapy are those with a wide QRS complex, HF, and impaired left ventricular function [47]. Biventricular pacing was first introduced in the early 1990s by Bakker et al. and Cazeau et al. [48, 49]. CRT with the ability to work as an ICD is termed CRT-D, whereas the term used for a CRT that solely has a pacing function is CRT-P.

4.1 Cardiac dyssynchrony

The dyssynchrony that is targeted with CRT is caused by delays in electrical conduction, and the main way to identify this is by assessing the QRS duration (in particular LBBB) [50]. A prolonged QRS duration has been associated with decreased LVEF [51]. In patients with HF, prolongation of the QRS complex has been shown to be an independent predictor of increased total mortality and SCD. LBBB is related to worse survival but not sudden death [52]. Partially, the mechanism behind dyssynchrony is prolongation of the AV interval, leading to late systolic contraction which may take the place of early diastolic filling as well as cause mitral regurgitation. Furthermore, conduction delays between and in the ventricles themselves result in asynchronous contraction in the left ventricular walls with subsequent loss of cardiac efficiency [9]. Long-standing cardiac dyssynchrony can result in remodeling of the heart, causing dilation of the left ventricle, deteriorating diastolic and systolic function and worsening of HF [53].

4.2 Important trials

Several trials have been conducted in order to optimize indications for CRT. The COmparison of Medical Therapy, Pacing and Defibrillation in Heart Failure (COMPANION) trial compared optimal medical therapy, CRT-D, and CRT-P, and found that all-cause mortality and hospitalization was reduced in both CRT groups. Reduction in mortality was however only marginally significant with CRT-P, but significant in the CRT-D group [54]. In the CArdiac REsynchronization in Heart Failure (CARE-HF) trial, optimal medical therapy was compared to CRT-P, with the result that CRT-P reduced all-cause mortality and hospitalization as well as improved symptoms and quality of life [55]. Both of these trials enrolled patients in NYHA class III-IV with a QRS duration of 120 ms or more. The Resynchronization-Defibrillation for Ambulatory Heart Failure Trial (RAFT) compared the rate of all-cause mortality and hospitalization due to HF between patients in NYHA class II or III with a QRS duration of at least 120 ms, randomized to either CRT-D or ICD, finding a reduction in the primary outcome in the CRT-D group [56].

In the REsynchronization reVErses Remodeling in Systolic left vEntricular dysfunction (REVERSE) trial, patients with HF in NYHA class I and II were randomized to CRT (with or without defibrillator) or control. The results showed an improvement in the ventricular structure and function in the CRT group and a decrease in hospitalization for HF [57]. MADIT-CRT was designed to evaluate the effect on death and HF events in patients in NYHA class I-II who received a CRT-D compared to an ICD. The risk of HF events was reduced, left ventricular volumes were reduced, and EF improved in the CRT-D group, but no significant difference in all-cause mortality was seen between the groups [58]. When the outcomes in MADIT-CRT were studied in relationship to whether or not the patient had LBBB, CRT-D led to a reduction in HF progression and a reduced risk of ventricular tachyarrhythmias in patients with LBBB while patients with non-LBBB morphology did not benefit clinically [59].

4.3 General indications for CRT

4.3.1 Patients in sinus rhythm

CRT is recommended by the ESC (class I recommendation) in patients with symptomatic HF in sinus rhythm, with a QRS duration of 130 ms or more, LBBB morphology, and an LVEF of 35% or less despite optimal medical therapy, to reduce symptoms, morbidity, and mortality [60]. CRT should be considered (class IIa recommendation) in patients who meet these criteria but do not have LBBB morphology and have a QRS duration of 150 ms or more and may be considered (class IIb recommendation) in non-LBBB morphology if the QRS duration is between 130 and 149 ms [60]. Patients with HF with reduced EF in any NYHA class who have an indication for bradycardia pacing with a high proportion of right ventricular pacing (high degree AV block, permanent AF) should receive CRT instead of a conventional pacemaker in order to reduce morbidity (class I recommendation) [60]. Lastly, patients with HF with reduced EF who already have a pacemaker or ICD and develop worsening HF despite optimal medical therapy and have a high rate of ventricular pacing may be considered for upgrade to CRT [60].

Since there have been few patients included in RCTs who are in NYHA class I or IV, the evidence for CRT in these patients is inconclusive. When it comes to NYHA class IV, individual consideration should be made. The recommendations from the ESC include patients in NYHA class IV who are ambulatory (no HF hospitalizations in the last month) [9].

4.3.2 Patients in atrial fibrillation

Since AF results in irregular and often fast ventricular rates, there is a risk that biventricular pacing delivery does not work adequately in these patients, and most of the patients with AF and an intact AV node require AV junction ablation in order for biventricular pacing to work properly. When considering AV junction ablation before CRT implantation, the risk that pacemaker dependency poses must of course be taken into account [9]. In its 2013 guidelines, the ESC suggests that CRT should be considered in patients with AF who have an EF of 35% or less, are in NYHA class III-IV despite optimal medical therapy, and have a QRS duration of at least 120 ms—provided that bi-ventricular capture of as close to 100% can be achieved. In case bi-ventricular pacing is incomplete, AV junction ablation should be performed [9]. CRT is not an indication for AV junction ablation in any other situation than when it is necessary because of consistently high ventricular rates despite optimal medical therapy [60]. In addition to this, CRT should be considered in patients with reduced EF who are candidates for AV junction ablation because of uncontrolled heart rate; a QRS duration of more than 120 ms is not necessary [9]. In the slightly more recent guidelines from 2016 regarding acute and chronic HF, a QRS duration of 130 ms is the cut off for when CRT is indicated (applies to patients in sinus rhythm as well as in AF) [60].

4.3.3 Patients with indications for bradycardia pacemakers

Right ventricular pacing might be associated with harmful effects on the cardiac function and structure; therefore, upgrading from a conventional pacemaker to CRT is recommended in patients with optimal medical therapy who have HF in NYHA class III and ambulatory class IV, EF of less than 35%, and a high percentage of right ventricular pacing [9]. It should be noted that upgrade to CRT implies a higher risk of complications compared to primary implantation [9]. In patients who have indications for bradycardia pacing and have not yet received a pacemaker, the ESC guidelines from 2013 recommend that CRT should be considered if they have a history of HF with reduced EF and an expected high rate of ventricular pacing in order to decrease the risk of worsening HF [9]. In its 2016 guidelines regarding acute and chronic HF, the ESC made CRT a class I recommendation (is recommended) in patients with HF with reduced EF regardless of NYHA class, who have an indication for ventricular pacing (patients with AF included) [60].

4.3.4 Patients with indications for ICD

Several studies, including the aforementioned RAFT and MADIT-CRT, that have compared ICD to CRT-D have found that CRT-D reduces morbidity and mortality. Therefore, when a patient is to receive an ICD, the presence of CRT indications (as mentioned) should be assessed [9]. According to the ESC guidelines, when ICD therapy is indicated in a HF patient who has a QRS complex duration between 130 and 149 ms, CRT-D should be considered. If the QRS duration is 150 ms or more, CRT-D is recommended [60].

4.3.5 The choice between CRT-P and CRT-D

In order to improve prognosis, evidence points toward the use of CRT-D therapy for patients in NYHA class II and CRT-P for patients in NYHA classes III-IV [60]. There is not sufficient evidence based on RCTs for the ESC to make a specific recommendation on when to choose one over the other, but they offer some advice. In addition to patients with advanced HF, the ESC suggests CRT-P in patients with severe renal insufficiency and those who have other major comorbidities, cachexia, or frailty. CRT-D, on the other hand, is more appropriate in patients with a life expectancy of at least a year, stable HF, no comorbidities, and ischemic heart disease [9].

4.4 Contraindications

According to the Echocardiography Guided Cardiac Resynchronization Therapy (EchoCRT) study, there is a risk of increased mortality when CRT is used in patients with systolic HF and a QRS duration of less than 130 [61]; QRS of less than 130 ms is therefore considered a contraindication to CRT by the ESC [60].

4.5 Cardiac contractility modulation

Patients who lack indications for CRT but still suffer from symptomatic HF with reduced EF in spite of optimal medical therapy might be candidates for cardiac contractility modulation (CCM). It provides nonexcitatory stimulation of the ventricle in its refractory period in order to improve contractility but not cause extra systolic contractions [60].

5. Future perspectives

An interesting area of research is the attempt to build biological pacemakers. Stem cells and viral vectors have been used to introduce ion-channel genes into the heart [62]. These preclinical attempts are promising but much remains until they are ready to be considered a clinical option [63]. Nevertheless, electronic devices have been developed over decades with proven efficacy, and devastating complications are rare.

Leadless pacing provides a landmark in the development of pacemaker technology. However, it is basically limited to pacing from the right ventricle. Because most patients will benefit from AV synchronization and even additional cardiac resynchronization, efforts are made to fulfill this demand. The AV-sequential challenge could potentially be solved by a VDD mode that would rely on atrial sensing from a subcutaneous integrated ECG device. Furthermore, device systems that are able to communicate between them are being developed. The subcutaneous ICD could be combined with a leadless pacemaker, which could provide sensing/pacing in the right ventricle, including antitachycardia pacing. The ultrasound-based technology WiCS™ system for endocardial pacing of the left ventricle is another option that is currently being developed [64]. The energy is transmitted from a subcutaneous transmitter subcutaneously to a receiver in the endocardium. Leadless pacing in the right ventricular chamber combined with the left-ventricular endocardial unit and a subcutaneous pulse generator could be a possibility in the near future.

6. Conclusions

Pacemaker therapy has revolutionized the treatment of bradycardia, and with an aging population, the use of permanent pacemakers is likely to increase. SCD, a major cause of death worldwide, can now be prevented with ICD therapy. CRT reduces symptoms and risk of death in patients who have HF with reduced EF and ventricular dyssynchrony. The indications for these therapies continue to evolve as new evidence emerges and novel technologies become available.

Conflict of interest

Peter Magnusson has received lecture fees from Abbott, Bayer, Boehringer-Ingelheim, Boston Scientific, Medtronic, MSD, Orion Pharma, and Pfizer.

Author details

Ida Åberg[1], Gustav Mattsson[1*] and Peter Magnusson[1,2]

1 Centre for Research and Development, Uppsala University, Gävle, Sweden

2 Cardiology Research Unit, Department of Medicine, Karolinska Institutet, Stockholm, Sweden

*Address all correspondence to: gustav.mattsson@regiongavleborg.se

References

[1] Aquilina O. A brief history of cardiac pacing. Images in Paediatric Cardiology. 2006;**8**(2):17-81

[2] Gregoratos G. Permanent pacemakers in older persons. Journal of the American Geriatrics Society. 1999;**47**(9):1125-1135

[3] Bradshaw PJ, Stobie P, Knuiman MW, Briffa TG, Hobbs MS. Trend in the incidence and prevalence of cardiac pacemaker insertions in an ageing population. Open Heart. 2014;**10**(1):e000177

[4] Gadler F, Valzania C, Linde C. Current use of implantable electrical devices in Sweden: Data from the Swedish pacemaker and implantable cardioverter-defibrillator registry. Europace. 2015;**17**(1):69-77

[5] Åberg I, Mattsson G, Magnusson P. Bradycardia: A clinician's guide to slow heart rates. EC Cardiology. 2018;**5**(6):316-325

[6] Mulpuru SK, Madhavan M, McLeod CJ, Cha YM, Friedman PA. Cardiac pacemakers: Function, troubleshooting, and management: Part 1 of a 2-part series. Journal of the American College of Cardiology. 2017;**69**(2):189-210

[7] Dell'Orto S, Valli P, Greco EM. Sensors for rate responsive pacing. Indian Pacing and Electrophysiology Journal. 2004;**4**(3):137-145

[8] Link MS, Hellkamp AS, Estes NA III, Orav EJ, Ellenbogen KA, Greenspon A, et al. High incidence of pacemaker syndrome in patients with sinus node dysfunction treated with ventricular-based pacing in the mode selection trial (MOST). Journal of the American College of Cardiology. 2004;**43**(11):2066-2071

[9] Brignole M, Auricchio A, Baron-Esquivias G, Bordachar P, Boriani G, Breithardt OA, et al. 2013 ESC guidelines on cardiac pacing and cardiac resynchronization therapy: The task force on cardiac pacing and resynchronization therapy of the European Society of Cardiology (ESC). Developed in collaboration with the European Heart Rhythm Association (EHRA). Europace. 2013;**15**(8):1070-1118

[10] Epstein AE, DiMarco JP, Ellenbogen KA, Estes NA III, Freedman RA, Gettes LS, et al. 2012 ACCF/AHA/HRS focused update incorporated into the ACCF/AHA/HRS 2008 guidelines for device-based therapy of cardiac rhythm abnormalities: A report of the American College of Cardiology Foundation/American Heart Association Task Force on Practice Guidelines and the Heart Rhythm Society. Journal of the American College of Cardiology. 2013;**61**(3):e6-e75

[11] Brubaker PH, Kitzman DW. Chronotropic incompetence: Causes, consequences, and management. Circulation. 2011;**123**(9):1010-1020

[12] Nielsen JC, Thomsen PE, Højberg S, Møller M, Vesterlund T, Dalsgaard D, et al. A comparison of single-lead atrial pacing with dual-chamber pacing in sick sinus syndrome. European Heart Journal. 2011;**32**(6):686-696

[13] Connolly SJ, Kerr CR, Gent M, Roberts RS, Yusuf S, Gillis AM, et al. Effects of physiologic pacing versus ventricular pacing on the risk of stroke and death due to cardiovascular causes. Canadian Trial of Physiologic Pacing Investigators. The New England Journal of Medicine. 2000;**342**(19):1385-1391

[14] Lamas GA, Lee KL, Sweeney MO, Silverman R, Leon A, Yee R, et al. Ventricular pacing or dual-chamber pacing for sinus-node dysfunction.

The New England Journal of Medicine. 2002;**346**(24):1854-1862

[15] Johansson BW. Longevity in complete heart block. Annals of the New York Academy of Sciences. 1969;**167**(2):1031-1037

[16] Toff WD, Camm AJ, Skehan JD. Single-chamber versus dual-chamber pacing for high-grade atrioventricular block. The New England Journal of Medicine. 2005;**353**(2):145-155

[17] Moya A, García-Civera R, Croci F, Menozzi C, Brugada J, Ammirati F, et al. Diagnosis, management, and outcomes of patients with syncope and bundle branch block. European Heart Journal. 2011;**32**(12):1535-1541

[18] Reddy VY, Knops RE, Sperzel J, Miller MA, Petru J, Simon J, et al. Permanent leadless cardiac pacing: Results of the LEADLESS trial. Circulation. 2014;**129**(14):1466-1471

[19] Duray GZ et al. Long-term performance of a transcatheter pacing system: 12-month results from the Micra Transcatheter Pacing Study. Heart Rhythm. 2017;**14**(5):702-709

[20] Neumar RW, Otto CW, Link MS, Kronick SL, Shuster M, Callaway CW, et al. Part 8: Adult advanced cardiovascular life support: 2010 American Heart Association Guidelines for Cardiopulmonary Resuscitation and Emergency Cardiovascular Care. Circulation. 2010;**122**:S729-S767

[21] Bektas F, Soyuncu S. The efficacy of transcutaneous cardiac pacing in ED. The American Journal of Emergency Medicine. 2016;**34**(11):2090-2093

[22] Gammage MD. Temporary cardiac pacing. Heart. 2000;**83**(6):715-720

[23] Mirowski M, Reid PR, Mower MM, Watkins L, Gott VL, Schauble JF, et al. Termination of malignant ventricular arrhythmias with an implanted automatic defibrillator in human beings. The New England Journal of Medicine. 1980;**303**(6):322-324

[24] Glikson M, Friedman PA. The implantable cardioverter defibrillator. Lancet. 2001;**357**(9262):1107-1117

[25] Priori SG, Blomström-Lundqvist C, Mazzanti A, Blom N, Borggrefe M, Camm J, et al. 2015 ESC guidelines for the management of patients with ventricular arrhythmias and the prevention of sudden cardiac death: The Task Force for the Management of Patients with Ventricular Arrhythmias and the Prevention of Sudden Cardiac Death of the European Society of Cardiology (ESC). European Heart Journal. 2015;**36**(41):2793-2867

[26] Huikuri HV, Castellanos A, Myerburg RJ. Sudden death due to cardiac arrhythmias. The New England Journal of Medicine. 2001;**345**(20):1473-1482

[27] Link MS, Atkins DL, Passman RS, Halperin HR, Samson RA, White RD, et al. Part 6: Electrical therapies: Automated external defibrillators, defibrillation, cardioversion, and pacing: 2010 American Heart Association Guidelines for Cardiopulmonary Resuscitation and Emergency Cardiovascular Care. Circulation. 2010;**122**:706-719

[28] Schaumann A, von zur Mülen F, Herse B, Gonska BD, Kreuzer H. Empirical versus tested antitachycardia pacing in implantable cardioverter defibrillators: A prospective study including 200 patients. Circulation. 1998;**97**(1):66-74

[29] The Antiarrhythmics versus Implantable Defibrillators (AVID) Investigators. A comparison of antiarrhythmic-drug therapy with implantable defibrillators in patients

resuscitated from near-fatal ventricular arrhythmias. The New England Journal of Medicine. 1997;**337**(22):1576-1583

[30] Kuck KH, Cappato R, Rüppel R. Randomized comparison of antiarrhythmic drug therapy with implantable defibrillators in patients resuscitated from cardiac arrest: The Cardiac Arrest Study Hamburg (CASH). Circulation. 2000;**102**(7):748-754

[31] Connolly SJ, Gent M, Roberts RS, Dorian P, Roy D, Sheldon RS, et al. Canadian implantable defibrillator study (CIDS): A randomized trial of the implantable cardioverter defibrillator against amiodarone. Circulation. 2000;**101**(11):1297-1302

[32] Connolly SJ, Hallstrom AP, Cappato R, Schron EB, Kuck KH, Zipes DP, et al. Meta-analysis of the implantable cardioverter defibrillator secondary prevention trials. AVID, CASH and CIDS studies. Antiarrhythmics vs Implantable Defibrillator study. Cardiac Arrest Study Hamburg. Canadian Implantable Defibrillator Study. European Heart Journal. 2000;**21**(24):2071-2078

[33] Mehta RH, Yu J, Piccini JP, Tcheng JE, Farkouh ME, Reiffel J, et al. Prognostic significance of postprocedural sustained ventricular tachycardia or fibrillation in patients undergoing primary percutaneous coronary intervention (from the HORIZONS-AMI Trial). The American Journal of Cardiology. 2012;**109**(6):805-812

[34] Brugada J, Campuzano O, Arbelo E, Sarquella-Brugada G, Brugada R. Present status of Brugada syndrome: JACC state-of-the-art review. Journal of the American College of Cardiology. 2018;**72**(9):1046-1059

[35] Bardy GH, Lee KL, Mark DB, Poole JE, Packer DL, Boineau R, et al. Amiodarone or an implantable cardioverter–defibrillator for congestive heart failure. New England Journal of Medicine. 2005;**352**(3):225-237

[36] Køber L, Thune JJ, Nielsen JC, Haarbo J, Vidbæk L, Korup E, et al. Defibrillator implantation in patients with nonischemic systolic heart failure. The New England Journal of Medicine. 2016;**375**(13):1221-1230

[37] Moss AJ, Hall WJ, Cannom DS, Daubert JP, Higgins SL, Klein H, et al. Improved survival with an implanted defibrillator in patients with coronary disease at high risk for ventricular arrhythmia. The New England Journal of Medicine. 1996;**335**(26):1933-1940

[38] Moss AJ, Zareba W, Hall WJ, Klein H, Wilber DJ, Cannom DS, et al. Prophylactic implantation of a defibrillator in patients with myocardial infarction and reduced ejection fraction. The New England Journal of Medicine. 2002;**346**(12):877-883

[39] Hohnloser SH, Kuck KH, Dorian P, Roberts RS, Hampton JR, Hatala R, et al. Prophylactic use of an implantable cardioverter–defibrillator after acute myocardial infarction. The New England Journal of Medicine. 2004;**351**(24):2481-2488

[40] Kadish A, Dyer A, Daubert JP, Quigg R, Estes NA, Anderson KP, et al. Prophylactic defibrillator implantation in patients with nonischemic dilated cardiomyopathy. The New England Journal of Medicine. 2004;**350**(21):2151-2158

[41] Reek S, Burri H, Roberts PR, Perings C, Epstein AE, Klein HU, et al. The wearable cardioverter-defibrillator: Current technology and evolving indications. Europace. 2017;**19**(3):335-345

[42] DiMarco JP. Implantable cardioverter–defibrillators. The New England Journal of Medicine. 2003;**349**(19):1836-1847

[43] Magyar-Russell G, Thombs BD, Cai JX, Baveja T, Kuhl EA, Singh PP, et al. The prevalence of anxiety and depression in adults with implantable cardioverter defibrillators: A systematic review. Journal of Psychosomatic Research. 2011;**71**(4):223-231

[44] Schron EB, Exner DV, Jenkins LS, Steinberg JS, Cook JR, Kutalek SP, et al. Quality of life in the antiarrhythmics versus implantable defibrillators trial: Impact of therapy and influence of adverse symptoms and defibrillator shocks. Circulation. 2002;**105**(5):589-594

[45] Morken IM, Bru E, Norekvål TM, Larsen AI, Idsoe T, Karlsen B, et al. Perceived support from healthcare professionals, shock anxiety and post-traumatic stress in implantable cardioverter defibrillator recipients. Journal of Clinical Nursing. 2014;**23**(3-4):450-460

[46] Abraham WT, Fisher WG, Smith AL, Delurgio DB, Leon AR, Loh E, et al. Cardiac resynchronization in chronic heart failure. The New England Journal of Medicine. 2002;**346**(24):1845-1853

[47] Leyva F, Nisam S, Auricchio A. 20 years of cardiac resynchronization therapy. Journal of the American College of Cardiology. 2014;**64**(10):1047-1058

[48] Bakker PF, Meijburg HW, de Vries JW, Mower MM, Thomas AC, Hull ML, et al. Biventricular pacing in end-stage heart failure improves functional capacity and left ventricular function. Journal of Interventional Cardiac Electrophysiology. 2000;**4**(2):395-404

[49] Cazeau S, Ritter P, Bakdach S, Lazarus A, Limousin M, Henao L, et al. Four chamber pacing in dilated cardiomyopathy. Pacing and Clinical Electrophysiology. 1994;**17**(11 Pt 2): 1974-1979

[50] Kass DA. Cardiac resynchronization therapy. Journal of Cardiovascular Electrophysiology. 2005;**16**(s1):S35-S41

[51] Murkofsky RL, Dangas G, Diamond JA, Mehta D, Schaffer A, Ambrose JA. A prolonged QRS duration on surface electrocardiogram is a specific indicator of left ventricular dysfunction [see comment]. Journal of the American College of Cardiology. 1998;**32**(2):476-482

[52] Iuliano S, Fisher SG, Karasik PE, Fletcher RD, Singh SN. QRS duration and mortality in patients with congestive heart failure. American Heart Journal. 2002;**143**(6):1085-1091

[53] Jaffe LM, Morin DP. Cardiac resynchronization therapy: History, present status, and future directions. The Ochsner Journal. 2014;**14**(4):596-607

[54] Bristow MR, Saxon LA, Boehmer J, Krueger S, Kass DA, De Marco T, et al. Cardiac-resynchronization therapy with or without an implantable defibrillator in advanced chronic heart failure. The New England Journal of Medicine. 2004;**350**(21):2140-2150

[55] Cleland JG, Daubert JC, Erdmann E, Freemantle N, Gras D, Kappenberger L, et al. The effect of cardiac resynchronization on morbidity and mortality in heart failure. The New England Journal of Medicine. 2005;**352**(15):1539-1549

[56] Tang AS, Wells GA, Talajic M, Arnold MO, Sheldon R, Connolly S, et al. Cardiac-resynchronization therapy for mild-to-moderate heart failure. The New England Journal of Medicine. 2010;**363**(25):2385-2395

[57] Linde C, Abraham WT, Gold MR, St John Sutton M, Ghio S, Daubert C, et al. Randomized trial of cardiac resynchronization in mildly symptomatic heart failure patients and in asymptomatic patients with left ventricular dysfunction and previous heart failure symptoms. Journal of the American College of Cardiology. 2008;**52**(23):1834-1843

[58] Moss AJ, Hall WJ, Cannom DS, Klein H, Brown MW, Daubert JP, et al. Cardiac-resynchronization therapy for the prevention of heart-failure events. The New England Journal of Medicine. 2009;**361**(14):1329-1338

[59] Zareba W, Klein H, Cygankiewicz I, Hall WJ, McNitt S, Brown M, et al. Effectiveness of cardiac resynchronization therapy by QRS morphology in the multicenter automatic defibrillator implantation trial-cardiac resynchronization therapy (MADIT-CRT). Circulation. 2011;**123**(10):1061-1072

[60] Ponikowski P, Voors AA, Anker SD, Bueno H, Cleland JGF, Coats AJS, et al. 2016 ESC guidelines for the diagnosis and treatment of acute and chronic heart failure: The task force for the diagnosis and treatment of acute and chronic heart failure of the European Society of Cardiology (ESC) developed with the special contribution of the Heart Failure Association (HFA) of the ESC. European Heart Journal. 2016;**37**(27):2129-2200

[61] Ruschitzka F, Abraham WT, Singh JP, Bax JJ, Borer JS, Brugada J, et al. Cardiac-resynchronization therapy in heart failure with a narrow QRS complex. The New England Journal of Medicine. 2013;**369**(15):1395-1405

[62] Rosen MR. Gene therapy and biological pacing. The New England Journal of Medicine. 2014;**371**(12):1158-1159

[63] Rosen MR, Robinson RB, Brink PR, Cohen IS. The road to biological pacing. Nature Reviews. Cardiology. 2011;**8**(11):656-666

[64] Sperzel J, Burri H, Gras D, Tjong FV, Knops RE, Hindricks G, et al. State of the art of leadless pacing. Europace. 2015;**17**(10):1508-1513

Chapter 3

The Subcutaneous Implantable Cardioverter-Defibrillator

Peter Magnusson, Joseph V. Pergolizzi and Jo Ann LeQuang

Abstract

The subcutaneous ICD (S-ICD) represents an important advancement in defibrillation therapy that obviates the need for a transvenous lead, the most frequent complication with transvenous devices. The S-ICD has been shown similarly safe and effective as transvenous ICD therapy, but the two devices are not interchangeable. The S-ICD is only suitable for patients who do not require bradycardia or antitachycardia pacing functionality. In patients with underlying diseases associated with polymorphic ventricular tachycardia and a long life expectancy, an S-ICD may be the preferred choice. Moreover, it is advantageous in the situation of increased risk of endocarditis, i.e., previous device system infection and immunosuppression, including hemodialysis. In patients with abnormal vascular access and/or right-sided heart structural abnormalities, it may be the only option. The S-ICD is bulkier, the battery longevity is shorter, and the device cost is higher, even though remote follow-up is possible. A two- or three-incision implant procedure has been described with a lateral placement of the device and a single subcutaneous lead. The rate of inappropriate therapy for both S-ICD and transvenous systems is similar, but S-ICD inappropriate shocks are more frequently attributable to oversensing, which can often be resolved with sensing adjustments.

Keywords: lead complications, subcutaneous ICD, sudden cardiac death, S-ICD, transvenous ICD, T-wave oversensing

1. Introduction

The subcutaneous implantable cardioverter defibrillator (S-ICD) offers an alternative rescue device for sudden cardiac death in the form of an implantable device that can offer defibrillation therapy without the need for a transvenous lead. Lead failure is the most frequent source of complication requiring surgical revision. Approximately 20% of transvenous leads fail within 10 years and extraction may lead to devastating complications, including death [1–5]. The S-ICD differs from conventional transvenous ICD systems in other important ways: an S-ICD requires no transvenous leads (the most frequent source of device complications) but S-ICDs do not offer bradycardia pacing, antitachycardia pacing, cardiac resynchronization, plus they have limited programmability. Approved in Europe in 2009, the S-ICD system (SQ-RX 1010, Boston Scientific, Natick, Massachusetts, USA) consists of a pulse generator and a tripolar defibrillation lead, both of which are implanted subcutaneously. In terms of size, weight, and footprint, the S-ICD device is larger and heavier than a conventional transvenous ICD (approximately 130 vs. 60 g, respectively).

S-ICDs are indicated for primary and secondary prevention but are seen as particularly useful for primary-prevention patients with a long life expectancy. The selection of an S-ICD system over a transvenous ICD may be based on a variety of factors. Transvenous ICD patients who experience device-related complications, such as lead problems, may be revised to an S-ICD device. In a German multicenter study, 25% of S-ICD patients had a previous transvenous system explanted because of device complications [6].

2. Implant techniques and considerations

The S-ICD system is composed of a tripolar parasternal lead, positioned to the left (about 1–2 cm) and parallel to the sternal midline; this lead plugs into the pulse generator, which is implanted over the fifth to sixth rib and positioned submuscularly between the midaxillarly and anterior axillary lines. The lead has three electrodes, two of which sense only. The defibrillation electrode is positioned between the two sensing electrodes. The sensing vector is created from the sensing electrode to the can, with the device automatically selecting the better electrode for the vector to assure optimal sensing. Device implantation may require minimal (to verify final position) to no fluoroscopy, as much of the technique relies on anatomical landmarks [7]. See **Figure 1**.

A three-incision technique (plus pocket formation) was originally pioneered for S-ICD implantation, and a newer two-incision approach has been described in the literature [8]. The two-incision approach creates an intermuscular pocket for the pulse generator rather than a subcutaneous pocket by incising the inframammary crease at the anterior border of the latissimus dorsi, allowing the generator to fit between the two muscles. Then a small incision at the xiphoid process (in the same direction as pocket incision) allows an electrode insertion device to tunnel the lead in place [8, 9]. In a study of 36 patients, the two-incision approach was found to be safe and effective and it may produce superior cosmetic results compared to the three-incision approach [9]. See **Figure 2**.

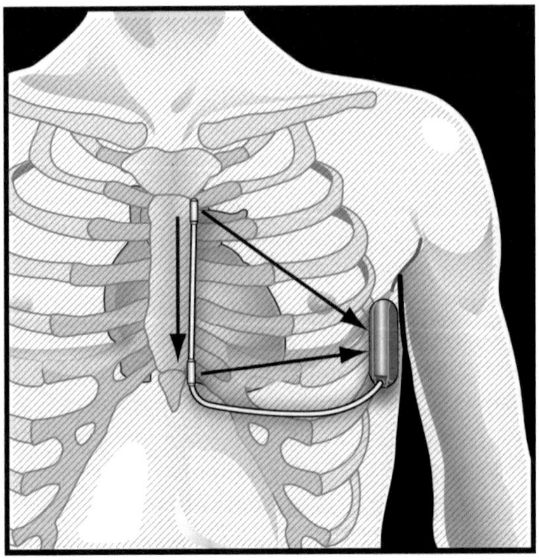

Figure 1.
The S-ICD device is implanted over the fifth to sixth rib and to the side; the parasternal lead senses the subcutaneous ECG and automatically determines which of two sensing vectors to use (top or bottom electrode to can). (Artwork by Todd Cooper, courtesy of Jo Ann LeQuang).

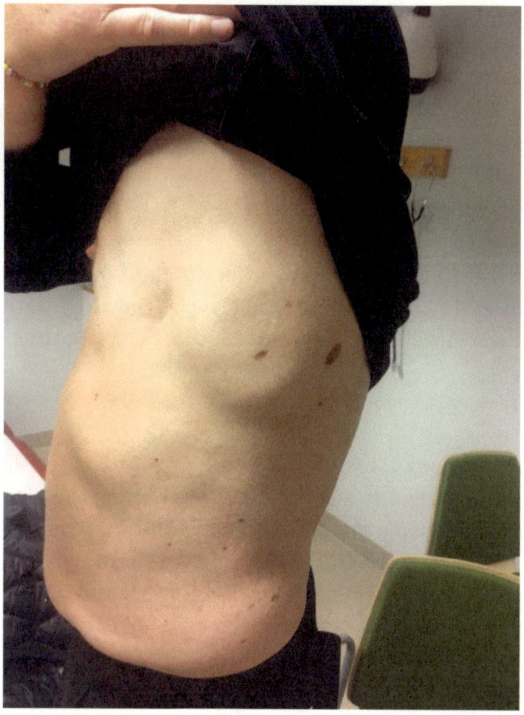

Figure 2.
Lateral view of a patient with an implanted S-ICD. (Courtesy of Dr. Peter Magnusson with permission of patient.).

The time required for device implantation has been recently reported as an average of 68 ± 20 minutes which includes intraoperative defibrillation threshold (DT) testing [10]. DT testing is of decreasing importance with transvenous ICDs but remains a much-discussed topic for S-ICD systems. Guidelines still recommend DT testing during S-ICD implantation, even though it is often used without intraoperative testing based on generalized findings from transvenous systems [11–13]. In a study of 98 S-ICD patients, 25% of patients failed to convert their induced arrhythmia with the first intraoperative 65 joule shock, necessitating further therapy delivery and/or external defibrillation. In this study, 24/25 patients could be successfully defibrillated following either reversal of shocking polarity or lead reposition although the desired 10 joules safety margin could not be achieved in 4/24 of these patients [14]. This suggests the importance of perioperative DT testing. However, 100% of patients could be converted from defibrillation with an internal 80 joule shock [14]. In a subsequent study of 110 consecutive S-ICD patients, 50% (n = 55) did not undergo defibrillation testing at implant for any of several reasons (including patient condition, age, and physician preference). In this group, 11% had episodes of sustained ventricular tachycardia (VT) or ventricular fibrillation (VF) necessitating therapy delivery and all of them were effectively converted with the first 80 joule shock [15]. Ventricular tachycardia is a rhythm disorder originating in the heart's lower chambers that has a rate of at least 100 beats per minute; ventricular fibrillation is a much faster, chaotic heart rhythm that causes the heart to quiver rather than pump effectively. Thus, the notion that DT testing at implant is necessary for S-ICD patients has been challenged.

S-ICD implantation may be carried out under local anesthesia [16], conscious sedation, or general anesthesia (64.1% of U.S. implants of S-ICD systems [17]. The rate of complications at implant is low and the most commonly reported complication is infection (1.8%) [18]. By dispensing with the transvenous leads, the S-ICD system avoids periprocedural and complications associated with conventional transvenous defibrillation leads, i.e. pericardial effusion, pneumothorax, accidental arterial puncture, nerve plexus injury, and tricuspid valve damage [19].

3. Safety and efficacy of S-ICDs

S-ICDs appear to have similar rates of infection and other complications as transvenous systems and to be similarly effective in rescuing patients from sudden cardiac death, but there are important distinctions between the two systems.

3.1 Safety

In a retrospective study of 1160 patients who received an implantable defibrillator (either transvenous system or S-ICD) at two centers in the Netherlands, patients were analyzed using propensity matching to yield 140 matched patient pairs. The rates of complications, infection, and inappropriate therapy were statistically similar between groups, but S-ICD patients had significantly fewer lead-related complications than the transvenous group (0.8 vs. 11.5%, $p = 0.030$) and more non-lead-related complications (9.9 vs. 2.2%, $p = 0.047$) [20]. The most frequently reported S-ICD complication involved device sensing.(20) Pooled data from the Investigational Device Exemption (IDE) and postmarket registry EFFORTLESS ($n = 882$) found S-ICD-related complications occurred at a rate of 11.1% at 3 years, but with no lead failures, S-ICD-related endocarditis, or bacteremia [21]. An IDE allows a device that is the subject of a clinical study to be used to collect data about safety and effectiveness that may be later used to submit to the U.S. Food and Drug Administration (FDA). Device-related complications were more frequent with transvenous systems when compared to S-ICD devices in a propensity-matched case–control study of 69 S-ICD and 69 transvenous ICD patients followed for a mean of 31 ± 19 or 32 ± 21 months, respectively. About 29% of transvenous ICD patients experienced a device-related complication compared to 6% of S-ICD patients, reducing the risk of complications for S-ICD patients by 70%; transvenous lead problems were the most frequently reported complication in the former group [22].

In the largest study of S-ICD patients ($n = 3717$) to date, complications were low at 1.2% overall. The most frequently reported complications were cardiac arrest (0.4%), hematoma (0.3%), death (0.3%), lead dislodgement (0.1%), myocardial infarction (0.1%), and hemothorax (<0.1%) [23]. Device revision during index hospitalization was infrequent (0.1%) [23]. Infections occur at roughly similar rates with S-ICD and transvenous systems but with the important distinction that S-ICD infections may sometimes be resolved with conservative therapy (course of antibiotics with device left in place), whereas most transvenous ICD infections necessitate the extraction of the device and the transvenous leads. In a survey from the U.K. reporting on data from 111 S-ICD patients, 11/111 (10%) of patients experienced infection, of whom 6 could be successfully treated conservatively without device extraction [24]. The EFFORTLESS registry ($n = 472$) reported a 4% rate of documented or suspected infections and complication-free rates at 30 and 360 days were 97 and 94%, respectively [25].

Once implanted, the S-ICD device delivers a nonprogrammable, high-energy rescue shock (80 joules) to the thorax compared to shocks of 45 joules to the heart administered by conventional transvenous systems. Notably the S-ICD delivers a 65 joule shock during implant testing. Therapy delivery differs markedly between S-ICD and transvenous systems in terms of the amount of energy delivered, location of shocking vectors, and potential for damage to surrounding tissue or the heart. In a porcine study, the mean time to therapy delivery was significantly longer with an S-ICD than a transvenous system (19 vs. 9 seconds, p = 0.001) but the S-ICD shocks were associated with less elevation of cardiac biomarkers. The longer time to therapy may be advantageous in that device patients often experience short runs of non-sustained VT. On the other hand, S-ICD shocks were associated with more skeletal muscle injuries than transvenous device shocks owing to the energy patterns resulting from the device placement but the clinical relevance of this is likely negligible [26].

3.2 Efficacy

Effective shock therapy is often defined as conversion of an episode of VT/VF within five shocks, differing from effective first-shock therapy which occurs when the initial shock converts the arrhythmia. In a study of 79 S-ICD patients at a tertiary center, 7.6% of patients experienced at least one appropriate shock for a ventricular tachyarrhythmia during the follow-up period (mean 12.8 ± 13.7 months) [27]. In a multicenter study from Germany (n = 40), shock efficacy was 96.4% [95% confidence interval (CI), 12.8–100%] and first-shock efficacy was 57.9% (95% CI, 35.6–77.4%) [6]. In an effort to analyze S-ICD efficacy in a large group of diverse patients, data from the Investigation Device Exemption (IDE) clinical study and the EFFORTLESS post-market registry were pooled to provide information about 882 patients followed for 651 ± 345 days. About 59 patients experienced therapy delivery for 111 spontaneous VT/VF episodes with first-shock efficacy in 90.1% of events and shock efficacy (termination with five or fewer shocks) in 98.2% of patients [21]. In the EFFORTLESS registry (n = 472), first-shock efficacy in discrete episodes of VT/VF was 88% and shock efficacy within five shocks was 100% [25].

4. Inappropriate shocks with S-ICDs

Inappropriate shock describes therapy delivery to treat an episode which the device inappropriately detects as a ventricular tachyarrhythmia. Inappropriate shocks have been recognized as a significant clinical challenge with transvenous systems as well as S-ICDs. In a tertiary care center study of 79 S-ICD patients, inappropriate shock occurred in 8.9% (n = 7) of patients, attributable to T-wave oversensing, atrial tachyarrhythmia with rapid atrioventricular conduction, external interference and/or baseline oversensing due to lead movement [27]. T-wave oversensing occurs when the device inappropriately senses ventricular repolarizations (the T-waves on the electrocardiograph) counting them as ventricular events, leading to double counting of the intrinsic ventricular rate. In a multicenter German study (n = 40) with a median follow-up of 229 days, four patients (10%) experienced 21 arrhythmic episodes resulting in 28 therapy deliveries. Four of these episodes were inappropriately identified by the device as ventricular tachyarrhythmias, with the result that two patients received inappropriate shocks. This results in a rate of 10% inappropriately detected ventricular tachycardia and 5% delivery of inappropriate therapy [6]. In a study using pooled data from the IDE and EFFORTLESS post-market registry (n = 882), the three-year rate for inappropriate therapy delivery was 13.1% [21].

It does not appear there are statistically more cases of inappropriate therapy in S-ICD patients compared to transvenous ICD patients. A propensity-matched study (69 patients with a transvenous ICD and 69 with an S-ICD) found the rate of inappropriate shocks was 9% in the transvenous and 3% in the S-ICD groups but this was not statistically significant (p = 0.49) [22]. In a study of 54 S-ICD patients in a real-world prospective registry, the one-year rate for inappropriate therapy delivery was 17%, most of whom had single-zone programming [10].

Inappropriate shocks with S-ICDs may be minimized. Most of them are caused by T-wave oversensing. In a survey from the U.K. (n = 111 implanted patients covered), 24 appropriate shocks were delivered in 12% of the patients (n = 13) and 51 inappropriate shocks were delivered in 15% of the patients (n = 17), of which 80% could be traced to T-wave oversensing [24]. In the EFFORTLESS registry (n = 472), there was a 7% rate of inappropriate therapy delivery in 360 days, mainly due to oversensing [25]. The main causes of inappropriate therapy delivery have been reported to be supraventricular tachycardia (SVT) at a rate above the discrimination zone, T-wave oversensing, other types of oversensing (e.g. interference), SVT discrimination errors, and low-amplitude signals [21]. Inappropriate therapy delivery due to T-wave oversensing can often be remedied by adjusting the sensing vector or adding another discrimination zone (dual-zone programming) [10].

Certain patients may be at elevated risk for inappropriate shock. A single-center study of 18 hypertrophic cardiomyopathy (HCM) patients implanted with an S-ICD system and followed for a mean 31.7 ± 15.4 months concluded that HCM patients may be at elevated risk for T-wave oversensing which could lead to inappropriate therapy delivery. In this study, 39% of these HCM patients had T-wave oversensing and 22% of the study population (n = 4) experienced inappropriate therapy delivery [28]. An evaluation of 581 S-ICD patients found that inappropriate shocks caused by oversensing occurred in 8.3% of S-ICD patients and patients with HCM and/or a history of atrial fibrillation were at elevated risk for inappropriate therapy [29]. There is a paucity of data on the use of S-ICD devices in HCM patients, but a small study of 27 HCM patients screened for possible S-ICD therapy found 85% (n = 23) were deemed appropriate candidates and 15 had the device implanted [30]. At implant testing, all patients were successfully defibrillated with a 65 joules shock and most induced arrhythmias were terminated with a 50 joules shock (12/15). After the median follow-up period of 17.5 months (range 3–35 months), there were no appropriate shocks and one inappropriate shock, attributed to oversensing caused when the QRS amplitude was reduced while the patient bent forward. In this particular high-risk patient group of HCM patients without a pacing indication, the S-ICD was effective at detecting and terminating tachyarrhythmias [30].

5. Mortality

The mortality risk with S-ICD implantation is low, but merits scrutiny. On the one hand, S-ICD implantation is generally associated with fewer risks than transvenous ICD implantation in that no transvenous leads are required. On the other hand, patient selection for S-ICD may favor more high-risk patients (such as those with a prior infection, renal failure, comorbid conditions such as diabetes) but also includes many younger and generally fitter patients. Overall, mortality data from S-ICD studies appears favorable. In a pooled analysis combining IDE data and EFFORTLESS registry information, the one-year and two-year mortality rates were 1.6 and 3.2%, respectively [21]. In a study of real-world use of S-ICDs in 54 primary- and secondary-prevention patients, mortality at the mean follow-up duration of 2.6 ± 1.9 years was 11% but no patient died of sudden cardiac arrest [10]. In a six-month study comparing 91 S-ICD and 182 single-chamber transvenous ICD patients, mortality rates were similar although the S-ICD patients had more severe pre-existing illness at implant [31]. It may be that the similar mortality rates between transvenous and S-ICD populations reflects the patient populations rather than the implantation procedure or device characteristics [23].

6. Troubleshooting S-ICDs

The S-ICD device was designed to be a streamlined system with fewer than 10 programmable features (transvenous ICDs have over 100 programmable features) and to perform in a largely automated fashion in terms of device function. The recent introduction of dual-zone programming to S-ICDs added a degree of programmability and reduced inappropriate shock [32]. Arrhythmia detection in the S-ICD relies on a system of template matching, based on waveform morphology of the subcutaneous ECG obtained at implant [33]. Oversensing and sensing-related problems are the most frequently reported problems but are being addressed in terms of device design and programmability. T-wave oversensing occurs when the device incorrectly identifies a T-wave as a QRS complex and counts it as a native ventricular beat, which leads to double-counting the rate. The use of dual-zone device programming has reduced the incidence of inappropriate therapy as a result of double-counting caused by T-wave oversensing [34]. T-wave inversions and QRS complexes that are overly large or very small may be particularly vulnerable to sensing anomalies. Reprogramming the sensing vector or therapy zones may be helpful in such instances [35, 36]. In a propensity-matched study comparing transvenous ICDs to S-ICDs, there were three inappropriate shocks in the S-ICD group, all of which were due to T-wave oversensing in sinus rhythm and all of which could be eliminated with adjustment of the sensing vector [22]. Furthermore, it has been observed with increasing operator experience and better programming techniques, sensing problems have been reduced [21]. In a study using pooled data from the IDE and EFFORTLESS registry, the rate of inappropriate therapy associated with oversensing was <1% [21]. When inappropriate shock occurs, the stored electrograms will likely help identify the cause. If lead malposition is suspected, a chest X-ray may be appropriate. In case of oversensing, the sensing vector may be optimized, device programming may be revised to add a second detection zone, or pharmacological therapy may be added [32].

SVT discrimination likewise relies on template matching (which is similar to transvenous systems) but the S-ICD may be able to accomplish this with a higher degree of resolution than transvenous ICDs [33]. The use of dual-zone programming appears advantageous.

7. Primary and secondary prevention

Primary- and secondary-prevention patients represent two distinct patient populations who may be treated with S-ICD therapy, although S-ICDs seem particularly well suited for primary-prevention patients. Secondary-prevention patients have a lower rate of comorbid conditions and significantly higher left-ventricular ejection fractions (LVEF) than primary-prevention patients (48 vs. 36%, $p < 0.0001$), while primary-prevention patients had a higher incidence of heart failure and were more likely to have had a transvenous ICD implanted before the S-ICD. Primary-prevention patients also have a higher rate of ischemic cardiomyopathy (41 vs. 33%) and nonischemic cardiomyopathy (28 vs. 12%) [18]. S-ICDs have been shown to be effective for both primary- and secondary-prevention patients. In a study of 856 S-ICD patients (mean follow-up 644 days), there were no significant differences between primary- and secondary-prevention populations in the rates of effective arrhythmia conversions, inappropriate therapy, mortality or complications although appropriate therapy delivery was delivered to significantly more secondary-prevention than primary prevention patients (11.9 vs. 5.0%, $p = 0.0004$) [18].

The freedom from any appropriate therapy delivery was 88.4% among primary-prevention patients with an LVEF ≤35 and 96.2% among primary-prevention patients with an LVEF >35%. The freedom from any appropriate therapy delivery among secondary-prevention patients was 92.1% [18]. Spontaneous conversion to sinus rhythm was more frequent among primary-prevention patients (about 48% of all ventricular tachyarrhythmias) compared to secondary-prevention patients (31%) [18]. However, the rates of inappropriate therapy delivery and complications were similar for both primary- and secondary-prevention patients [18].

8. The optimal candidates for S-ICD

S-ICD systems are indicated for patients who require rescue defibrillation but do not need bradycardia pacing support and would not benefit from antitachycardia pacing or cardiac resynchronization therapy. This includes primary- and secondary-prevention patients. By avoiding transvenous leads, the S-ICD is particularly appropriate for patients with occluded veins or limited venous access (who are not suitable candidates for transvenous systems) and the S-ICD may be beneficial for younger, fitter, and active patients. The generator position of the S-ICD patient may make it easier and safer for strong, fit patients to resume active lifestyles without jeopardizing lead position.

Despite the fact that S-ICD devices are larger than transvenous systems, their lateral placement may result in more pleasing esthetic results than a conventional transvenous ICD. Young device patients likely will have a lifetime of device therapy, resulting over time in much hardware in their vasculature; the S-ICD thus presents an advantage in that regard. It appears that S-ICDs are implanted in a younger patient population; a survey of multiple U.K. hospitals (n = 111 patients) found the median patient age was 33 (range 10–87 years) [24]. The mean age of patients in the EFFORTLESS registry was 49 ± 18 years (range 9–88 years) [25]. Younger patients with cardiomyopathy or channelopathy often have a high rate of complications with conventional transvenous ICDs [37] and it has been thought they may be better served with an S-ICD device [9].

In a multicenter case–control study, it was found that 59.4% of S-ICD patients were primary-prevention and the main underlying cardiac conditions were dilated cardiomyopathy (36.2%), ischemic cardiomyopathy (15.9%), and HCM (14.5%) [38]. In particular, these patients have been considered challenging to treat with a conventional transvenous ICD in that they may have an erratic electrical substrate in the heart and increased left-ventricular mass, which could contribute to an elevated DT. First-shock efficacy rates of up to 88% are promising in light of these challenges [25]. In a study of 50 hypertrophic cardiomyopathy patients implanted with S-ICDs, 96% of patients could be induced to an arrhythmia at implant and of the 73 episodes of VF induced, 98% were successfully converted with 65 joules from the S-ICD during DT testing. One patient in this study (2%) required rescue external defibrillation [39]. The patient who failed internal defibrillation had a body mass index of 36 and was successfully converted by an 80 joules shock with reversed polarity from the S-ICD [39].

9. Current guidelines

9.1 Indications

The most recent guidelines to address S-ICD were published by the American Heart Association, the American College of Cardiology, and the Heart Rhythm

Society in 2017 [40]. The An S-ICD is indicated (Class of Recommendation 1, level of evidence B) for patients who meet indication criteria for a transvenous ICD but who have inadequate vascular access or are at high risk of infection and for whom there is no anticipated need for bradycardia or antitachycardia pacing. Further, implantation of an S-ICD is deemed reasonable for patients with an ICD indication for whom there is no anticipated need for bradycardia or antitachycardia pacing (Class of Recommendation IIa, level of evidence B). An S-ICD is contraindicated in a patient who is indicated for bradycardia pacing, antitachycardia pacing for termination of ventricular tachyarrhythmias, and/or cardiac resynchronization therapy (Class of Recommendation III, level of evidence B) [40].

The European Society of Cardiology guidelines from 2015 report that S-ICDs are effective in preventing sudden cardiac death and the device is recommended as an alternative to transvenous ICDs in patients who are indicated for defibrillation but not pacing support, cardiac resynchronization therapy, or antitachycardia pacing (Class IIa, Level C). Moreover, the S-ICD was considered to be a useful alternative for patients in whom venous access was difficult or for patients who had a transvenous system explanted because of an infection or for young patients expected to need long-term ICD therapy [41].

9.2 Pre-implant testing

Those considered for S-ICD therapy should be screened with a modified version of the three-channel surface electrocardiogram (ECG) set up to represent the sensing vectors of the S-ICD. With the patient both standing and supine, the ratio of R-wave to T-wave should be established and signal quality evaluated. If any of the three vectors does not result in satisfactory sensing, the S-ICD should not be implanted. Once the actual device is implanted in the patient, the system automatically selects the optimal sensing vector [11].

9.3 Programming

The S-ICD may be programmed to detect arrhythmias using a single- or dual-zone configuration. In the dual-zone configuration, a lower cutoff rate defines what might be called a "conditional shock zone" to which a discrimination algorithm is applied so that therapy is withheld if the rhythm might be deemed supraventricular in origin or non-arrhythmic oversensing. This discrimination zone relies on a form of template matching. Above that rate, a cutoff establishes the "shock zone" which delivers a shock based on the rate criterion alone. When the capacitors charge in anticipation of shock delivery, a confirmation algorithm assures the persistence of the arrhythmia prior to sending the shock. Shocks are delivered at the nonprogrammable 80 joules of energy [11].

10. Future directions

The evolution of the S-ICD adds an important new device into the armamentarium for rescuing patients from sudden cardiac death. To further improve S-ICD technology, size reduction, increased battery longevity, and improved T-wave rejection will be needed. In the near future, improvement in sensing function might eliminate the need for a separate screening ECG prior to implant, which could optimize clinical workflow.

Improved battery technology is particularly important as the S-ICD is often used in patients with a relatively long life expectancy. Leadless pacemaker systems that might work together with an S-ICD are in development which would allow for bradycardia pacing support, antitachycardia pacing and a subcutaneous defibrillator without transvenous leads [32]. The development of a leadless epicardial pacemaker might allow for left-atrial and left-ventricular pacing function to be integrated to the S-ICD. Taken altogether, these improvements could make the S-ICD the preferred device in the vast majority of cases for rescue from sudden cardiac death.

11. Conclusion

The subcutaneous implantable cardioverter defibrillator (S-ICD) offers an alternative to transvenous ICDs but the two systems should not be considered interchangeable. The S-ICD is appropriate for patients who require only rescue defibrillation (primary or secondary prevention) but does not offer bradycardia pacing, antitachycardia pacing, overdrive pacing, or cardiac resynchronization therapy. S-ICD devices may be appropriate in patients who have occluded vasculature or device infection with a transvenous system. Effectiveness, rate of infections, and survival rates are similar for both devices although, in general, S-ICDs may be implanted in patients with more serious underlying conditions such as end-stage renal disease or advanced diabetes. Infections with S-ICDs are more likely to be effectively treated with a conservative course of antibiotic therapy and no device extraction. Inappropriate shocks occur at similar rates with both systems but are more likely caused by oversensing in the S-ICD. A main advantage of S-ICDs over transvenous systems is the elimination of the transvenous defibrillation lead which may be considered the Achilles heel of the transvenous system, having a 10-year complication rate of 25%. It is likely that considerable advances in ICD therapy will occur in the next decade as the S-ICD systems are further refined.

Conflict of interest

The authors have no conflicts of interest to declare.

Author details

Peter Magnusson[1,2], Joseph V. Pergolizzi[3] and Jo Ann LeQuang[4*]

1 Cardiology Research Unit, Department of Medicine, Karolinska Institute, Stockholm, Sweden

2 Centre for Research and Development, Uppsala University/Region Gävleborg, Sweden

3 Native Cardio, Inc., Naples, Florida, USA

4 NEMA Research Inc., Naples, Florida, USA

*Address all correspondence to: joann@leqmedical.com

References

[1] Kleemann T, Becker T, Doenges K, Vater M, Senges J, Schneider S, et al. Annual rate of transvenous defibrillation lead defects in implantable cardioverter-defibrillators over a period of >10 years. Circulation. 2007;**115**:2474-2480. DOI: 10.1161/CIRCULATIONAHA.106.663807

[2] Maisel WH, Kramer DB. Implantable cardioverter-defibrillator lead performance. Circulation. 2008;**117**:2721-2723. DOI: 10.1161/CIRCULATIONAHA.108.776807

[3] Alter P, Waldhans S, Plachta E, Moosdorf R, Grimm W. Complications of implantable cardioverter defibrillator therapy in 440 consecutive patients. Pacing and Clinical Electrophysiology: PACE. 2005;**28**:926-932. DOI: 10.1111/j.1540-8159.2005.00195.x

[4] Borleffs CJ, van Erven L, van Bommel RJ, van der Velde ET, van der Wall EE, Bax JJ, et al. Risk of failure of transvenous implantable cardioverter-defibrillator leads. Circulation. Arrhythmia and Electrophysiology. 2009;**2**:411-416. DOI: 10.1161/CIRCEP.108.834093

[5] Kalahasty G, Ellenbogen KA. Management of the patient with implantable cardioverter-defibrillator lead failure. Circulation. 2011;**123**:1352-1354. DOI: 10.1161/CIRCULATIONAHA.110.986828

[6] Aydin A, Hartel FW, Schluter M, Butter C, Kobe J, Seifert M, et al. Shock efficacy of subcutaneous implantable cardioverter-defibrillator for prevention of sudden cardiac death. Circulation. Arrhythmia and Electrophysiology. 2012;**5**:913-919. DOI: 10.1161/CIRCEP.112.973339

[7] Bardy GH, Smith WM, Hood MA, Crozier IG, Melton IC, Jordaens L, et al. An entirely subcutaneous implantable cardioverter-defibrillator. The New England Journal of Medicine. 2010;**363**:36-44. DOI: 10.1056/NEJMoa0909545

[8] Winter J, Siekiera M, Shin DI, Meyer C, Kropil P, Clahsen H, et al. Intermuscular technique for implantation of the subcutaneous implantable cardioverter defibrillator: Long-term performance and complications. Europace. 2017;**19**:2036-2041. DOI: 10.1093/europace/euw297

[9] Migliore F, Allocca G, Calzolari V, Crosato M, Facchin D, Daleffe E, et al. Intermuscular two-incision technique for subcutaneous implantable Cardioverter defibrillator implantation: Results from a multicenter registry. Pacing and Clinical Electrophysiology: PACE. 2017;**40**:278-285. DOI: 10.1111/pace.12987

[10] Mesquita J, Cavaco D, Ferreira A, Lopes N, Santos PG, Carvalho MS, et al. Effectiveness of subcutaneous implantable cardioverter-defibrillators and determinants of inappropriate shock delivery. International Journal of Cardiology. 2017;**232**:176-180. DOI: 10.1016/jicard.2017.01.034

[11] Wilkoff BL, Fauchier L, Stiles MK, Morillo CA, Al-Khatib SM, Almendral J, et al. 2015 HRS/EHRA/APHRS/SOLAECE expert consensus statement on optimal implantable cardioverter-defibrillator programming and testing. Europace. 2016;**18**:159-183. DOI: 10.1093/europace/euv411

[12] Bansch D, Bonnemeier H, Brandt J, Bode F, Svendsen JH, Taborsky M, et al. Intra-operative defibrillation testing and clinical shock efficacy in patients with implantable cardioverter-defibrillators: The NORDIC ICD randomized clinical trial. European Heart Journal. 2015;**36**:2500-2507. DOI: 10.1093/eurheartj/ehv292

[13] Healey JS, Hohnloser SH, Glikson M, Neuzner J, Mabo P, Vinolas X, et al. Cardioverter defibrillator implantation without induction of ventricular fibrillation: A single-blind, non-inferiority, randomised controlled trial (SIMPLE). Lancet. 2015;**385**(14):785, 61903-791, 61906. DOI: 10.1016/S01410-6736

[14] Frommeyer G, Zumhagen S, Dechering DG, Larbig R, Bettin M, Loher A, et al. Intraoperative defibrillation testing of subcutaneous implantable Cardioverter-defibrillator systems–A Simple issue. Journal of the American Heart Association. 2016;**5**:e003181. DOI: 10.1161/JAHA.115.003181

[15] Miller MA, Palaniswamy C, Dukkipati SR, Balulad S, Smietana J, Vigdor A, et al. Subcutaneous implantable cardioverter-defibrillator implantation without defibrillation testing. Journal of the American College of Cardiology. 2017;**69**:3118-3119. DOI: 10.1016/j.jacc.2017.04.037

[16] Dabiri Abkenari L, Theuns D, Valk S, Van Belle Y, de Groot N, Haitsma D, et al. Clinical experience with a novel subcutaenous implantable defibrillator system in a single center. Clinical Research in Cardiology: Official Journal of the German Cardiac Society. 2011;**100**:737-744. DOI: 10.1007/00392-011-0303-6

[17] Gold MR, Aasbo JD, El-Chami MF, Niebauer M, Herre J, Prutkin JM, et al. Subcutaneous implantable cardioverter-defibrillator post-approval study: Clinical characteristics and perioperative results. Heart Rhythm: The Official Journal of the Heart Rhythm Society. 2017;**14**:1456-1463. DOI: 10.1016/j.hrthm.2017.05.016

[18] Boersma LV, Barr CS, Burke MC, Leon AR, Theuns DA, Herre JM, et al. Performance of the subcutaneous implantable cardioverter-defibrillator in patients with a primary prevention indication with and without a reduced ejection fraction versus patients with a secondary prevention indication. Heart Rhythm: The Official Journal of the Heart Rhythm Society. 2017;**14**:367-375. DOI: 10.1016/j.hrthmj.2016.11.025

[19] Olde Nordkamp LRA, Conte G, Rosenmoller B, Warnaars JLF, Tan HL, Caputo ML, et al. Brugada syndrome and the subcutaneous implantable cardioverter-defibrillator. Journal of the American College of Cardiology. 2016;**68**:665-666. DOI: 10.1016/j.jacc.2016.05.058

[20] Brouwer TF, Yilmaz D, Lindeboom R, Buiten MS, Olde Nordkamp LR, Schalij MJ, et al. Long-term clinical outcomes of subcutaneous versus transvenous implantable defibrillator therapy. Journal of the American College of Cardiology. 2016;**68**:2047-2055. DOI: 10.1016/j.jacc.2016.08.044

[21] Burke MC, Gold MR, Knight BP, Barr CS, Theuns DA, Boersma LV, et al. Safety and efficacy of the totally subcutaneous implantable defibrillator: 2-year results from a pooled analysis of the IDE study and EFFORTLESS registry. Journal of the American College of Cardiology. 2015;**65**:1605-1615. DOI: 10.1016/j.jacc.2015.02.047

[22] Honarbakhsh S, Providencia R, Srinivasan N, Ahsan S, Lowe M, Rowland E, et al. A propensity matched case-control study comparing efficacy, safety and costs of the subcutaneous vs. transvenous implantable cardioverter defibrillator. International Journal of Cardiology. 2017;**228**:280-285. DOI: 10.1016/j.ijcard.2016.11.017

[23] Friedman DJ, Parzynski CS, Varosy PD, Prutkin JM, Patton KK, Mithani A, et al. Trends and in-hospital outcomes associated with adoption of the subcutaneous implantable cardioverter defibrillator in the United States. JAMA

Cardiology. 2016;**1**:900-911. DOI: 10.1001/jamacardio.2016.2782

[24] Jarman JW, Todd DM. United Kingdom national experience of entirely subcutaneous implantable cardioverter-defibrillator technology: Important lessons to learn. Europace. 2013;**15**:1158-1165. DOI: 10.1093/europace/eut016

[25] Lambiase PD, Barr C, Theuns DA, Knops R, Neuzil P, Johansen JB, et al. Worldwide experience with a totally subcutaneous implantable defibrillator: Early results from the EFFORTLESS S-ICD registry. European Heart Journal. 2014;**35**:1657-1665. DOI: 10.1093/eurheartj/ehu112

[26] Garcia R, Inal S, Favreau F, Jayle C, Hauet T, Bruneval P, et al. Subcutaneous cardioverter defibrillator has longer time to therapy but is less cardiotoxic than transvenous cardioverter defibrillator. Study carried out in a preclinical porcine model. Europace. 2018;**20**:873-879. DOI: 10.1093/europaceeux074

[27] Khazen C, Magnusson P, Flandorfer J, Schukro C. The subcutaneous implantable cardioverter-defibrillator: A tertiary center experience. Cardiology Journal. 2 May 2018. DOI: 10.5603/CJ.a2018.0050. [Epub ahead of print]

[28] Frommeyer G, Dechering DG, Zumhagen S, Loher A, Kobe J, Eckardt L, et al. Long-term follow-up of subcutaneous ICD systems in patients with hypertrophic cardiomyopathy: A single-center experience. Clinical Research in Cardiology: Official Journal of the German Cardiac Society. 2016;**105**:89-93. DOI: 10.1007/s00392-015-0901-9

[29] Olde Nordkamp LR, Brouwer TF, Barr C, Theuns DA, Boersma LV, Johansen JB, et al. Inappropriate shocks in the subcutaneous ICD: Incidence, predictors and management. International Journal of Cardiology. 2015;**195**:126-133. DOI: 10.1016/j.ijcard.2015.015.135

[30] Weinstock J, Bader YH, Maron MS, Rowin EJ, Link MS. Subcutaneous implantable cardioverter defibrillator in patients with hypertrophic cardiomyopathy: An initial experience. Journal of the American Heart Association. 2016;**5**:piie002488. DOI: 10.1161/JAHA.115.002488

[31] Mithani AA, Kath H, Hunter K, Andriulli J, Ortman M, Field J, et al. Characteristics and early clinical outcomes of patients undergoing totally subcutaneous vs. transvenous single chamber implantable cardioverter defibrillator placement. Europace. 2018;**20**:308-314. DOI: 10.1093/europace/eux026

[32] McLeod CJ, Boersma L, Okamura H, Friedman PA. The subcutaneous implantable cardioverter defibrillator: State-of-the-art review. European Heart Journal. 2017;**38**:247-257. DOI: 10.1093/eurheartj/ehv507

[33] De Maria E, Olaru A, Cappelli S. The entirely subcutaneous defibrillator (s-icd): State of the art and selection of the ideal candidate. Current Cardiology Reviews. 2015;**11**:180-186. DOI: 10.2174/157403X10666140827094126

[34] Weiss R, Knight BP, Gold MR, Leon AR, Herre JM, Hood M, et al. Safety and efficacy of a totally subcutaneous implantable-cardioverter defibrillator. Circulation. 2013;**128**:944-953. DOI: 10.1161/CIRCULATIONAHA.113.003042

[35] Gold MR, Theuns DA, Knight BP, Sturdivant JL, Sanghera R, Ellenbogen KA, et al. Head-to-head comparison of arrhythmia discrimination performance of subcutaneous and transvenous ICD arrhythmia detection algorithms: The START study. Journal of Cardiovascular Electrophysiology. 2012;**23**:359-366. DOI: 10.1111/j.1540-8167.2011.02199

[36] Kooiman KM, Knops RE, Olde Nordkamp L, Wilde AA, de Groot JR. Inappropriate subcutaneous implantable cardioverter-defibrillator shocks due to T-wave oversensing can be prevented: Implications for management. Heart Rhythm: The Official Journal of the Heart Rhythm Society. 2014;**11**:426-434. DOI: 10.1016/j.hrthm.2013.12.007

[37] Migliore F, Silvano M, Zorzi A, Bertaglia E, Siciliano M, Leoni L, et al. Implantable cardioverter defibrillator therapy in young patients with cardiomyopathies and channelopathies: A single Italian Centre experience. Journal of Cardiovascular Medicine (Hagerstown, Md). 2016;**17**:485-493. DOI: 10.2459/JCM.0000000000000395

[38] Kobe J, Reinke F, Meyer C, Shin DI, Martens E, Kaab S, et al. Implantation and follow-up of totally subcutaneous versus conventional implantable cardioverter-defibrillators: A multicenter case-control study. Heart Rhythm: The official Journal of the Heart Rhythm Society. 2013;**10**:29-36. DOI: 10.1016/j.hrthm.2012.09.126

[39] Maurizi N, Tanini I, Olivotto I, Amendola E, Limongelli G, Losi MA, et al. Effectiveness of subcutaneous implantable cardioverter-defibrillator testing in patients with hypertrophic cardiomyopathy. International Journal of Cardiology. 2017;**231**:115-119. DOI: 10.1016/j.ijcard.2016.12.187

[40] Al-Khatib SM, Stevenson WG, Ackerman MJ, Gillis AM, Bryant WJ, et al. AHA/ACC/HRS guideline for management of patients with ventricular arrhythmias and the prevention of sudden cardiac death: Executive summary: A report of the American College of Cardiology/American Heart Association task force on clinical practice guidelines and the Heart Rhythm Society. Heart Rhythm: The Official Journal of the Heart Rhythm Society. 30 Oct 2017. pii: **S1547-5271**(17);31249-31253. DOI: 10.1016/j.hrthm.2017.10.035. [Epub ahead of print] No abstract available. PMID: 29097320

[41] Priori SG, Blomstrom-Lundqvist C, Mazzanti A, Blom N, Borggrefe M, Camm J, et al. ESC guidelines for the management of patients with ventricular arrhythmias and the prevention of sudden cardiac death: The task force for the management of patients with ventricular arrhythmias and the prevention of sudden cardiac death of the European Society of Cardiology (ESC). Endorsed by: Association for European Paediatric and Congenital Cardiology (AEPC). European Heart Journal. 2015;**36**:2793-2867. DOI: 10.1093/eurheartj/ehv316

Chapter 4

Leadless Pacemakers

Peter Magnusson, Joseph V. Pergolizzi Jr and Jo Ann LeQuang

Abstract

Leadless or transcatheter pacemakers have recently been introduced to market with important benefits and some limitations. Implanted entirely within the right ventricle, these devices eliminate the need for transvenous pacing leads and pacemaker pockets and thus reduce the risk of infections and lead-related problems. Currently, they offer only VVI/R pacing and they cannot provide atrial sensing, antitachycardia pacing, or AV synchrony. They offer a number of features (such as rate response) and electrogram storage, albeit more limited than in a transvenous system. Real-world clinical data are needed to better comment on projected battery life, which manufacturers suggest will be at least equivalent to transvenous devices. Extracting an implanted leadless pacemaker remains a challenge, although proprietary snare and removal systems are available. However, a leadless pacemaker at end of service may be programmed to OOO and left in place; a revised device may be implanted adjacent. These innovative new devices may have important uses in special populations. Initial data on implant success and adverse events are favorable. Currently, there are two leadless pacemakers available: the Micra™ device by Medtronic and the Nanostim™ device by Abbott (formerly St. Jude Medical).

Keywords: LEADLESS clinical study, leadless pacemaker, Micra™ pacemaker, Nanostim™ pacemaker, transcatheter pacemaker

1. Introduction

The most vulnerable portion of the implantable cardiac pacemaker system is the transvenous lead(s), which can dislodge, fracture, experience insulation breach, and may lead to a host of adverse events including perforation, venous occlusion, tricuspid regurgitation, oversensing (with inappropriate device function), and infection. The innovation of a leadless pacemaker offers pacing support through a catheter-delivered device that is situated entirely within the right ventricle. A leadless pacemaker eliminates the need for both a pacemaker pocket and transvenous access. Its main limitations are lack of atrial pacing and sensing capabilities and the inability to provide antitachycardia pacing. For patients who require solely single-chamber ventricular pacing (VVI/R), the leadless pacemaker offers an important new option. Growing experience with these leadless devices shows great promise and expanding applications, even though real-world clinical experience is limited. The Spanish Pacemaker Registry reported about 1.6% leadless pacemakers out of all 12,697 reported devices by 2016 [1]. Despite this slow uptake, leadless pacing systems may be an important "disrupting technology" in cardiac rhythm management.

IntechOpen

2. Device description

There are currently two commercially available leadless pacemakers, which are designed to reside entirely within the right ventricle, affixed to the ventricular septum either mid-way or near the apex (see **Figure 1**). These devices are manufactured by two of the leading pacemaker companies in the world: Medtronic makes the Micra™ leadless pacemaker and Abbott (formerly St. Jude Medical) the Nanostim™ leadless pacemaker. The devices are cylindrical, attach directly to right ventricular septum, and have pacing and sensing electrodes that adhere to the myocardium with a retrieval loop on the other end of the device to facilitate extraction.

Leadless pacemakers are capable of pacing in the VVI mode with the programmable option of rate response (VVIR). The Medtronic device contains a lithium-silver-vanadium-oxide/carbon monofluoride battery (120 mAh), while the Abbott device utilizes a lithium carbon monofluoride battery with 248 mAh [2]. Both devices weigh about 2 g; the Abbott device (Nanostim™) is longer and thinner (42 mm in length and 5.99 mm diameter), while the Medtronic device (Micra™) is shorter and thicker (25.9 and, 6.7 mm) [2]. The Abbott device is secured via an active-fixation type helix mechanism, while the Medtronic device relies on passive fixation with nitinol tines [3]. Battery longevity in leadless pacemakers is estimated to be about 12–14 years. The Abbott (Nanostim™) leadless pacemaker was the subject of a global alert in late 2016 because of premature battery depletion that could result in loss of output and telemetry. The battery is a proprietary lithium-carbon monofluoride cell. Of 1423 Nanostim™ implantations around the world, 34 batteries failed (about 2%), but without any associated patient injury [4].

Leadless pacemakers at present cannot offer dual-chamber pacing modes or anti-tachycardia pacing; thus, they are only appropriate for patients who require VVI/VVIR or VOO/VOOR pacing. Electrogram storage is possible but there is limited device memory compared to transvenous pacemaker systems [5].

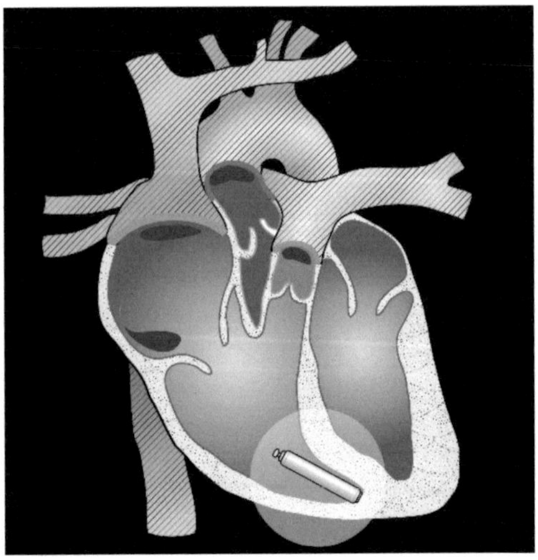

Figure 1.
The leadless pacemaker is implanted via a catheter into the right ventricle and affixed near the apex or midway on the right-ventricular septum where the operator attains acceptable electrical measurements (capture threshold, R-wave amplitude, and pacing impedance). The integral pacing and sensing electrodes in the device eliminate the need for transvenous pacing leads (illustration by Todd Cooper).

3. Implantation techniques

Leadless pacemakers are typically implanted via right or left femoral venous access into the septal wall of the right ventricle, although a right internal jugular vein approach has been described in the literature [6]. Right femoral access is preferred as the femoral iliac system nothing is less sharply angled on this side at the point where it joins the inferior vena cava [7]. The outer delivery sheath needed to deliver the pacemaker may have a diameter of 27 French (9 mm), which can be accommodated at implant by using a step-up sequence of dilators. Ultrasound with or without micropuncture has been recommended to avoid accidental arterial puncture or suboptimal sites of femoral puncture. As delivery sheaths may be large caliber, a poorly positioned puncture may make hemostasis challenging at the point when the sheath is withdrawn [7]. The proprietary delivery catheter is deflectable and advances with the device via the superior or inferior vena cava into the right atrium, over the tricuspid valve, and then into the right ventricle. The delivery catheter releases the device, which is affixed by active- or passive-fixation mechanisms to the endocardium [7]. Fluoroscopy may be used to confirm appropriate position. On radiography, the implanted devices look like a small cylinder (about the size and shape of a triple-A battery) [8]. Appropriate position is confirmed with acceptable electrical measurements generally defined as capture threshold ≤1.0 V at 0.24–0.4 ms, R-wave >6 mV, and impedance >500 Ω. The introducer sheath is then detached and removed and hemostasis achieved by a closure device, sutures, or manual pressure [7].

Unlike pacing thresholds with transvenous systems, which tend to gradually rise weeks after implant, the capture threshold for a leadless device may be expected to decrease somewhat about 30 min after implant and then stabilize. In two cases reports, threshold values in for a leadless pacemaker (Nanostim™) decreased markedly during the perioperative period. In one case, the pacing threshold was >6.5 V, the initial R-wave was >12.0 mV, and impedance was 1830 Ω. Rather than reposition the system, it was decided to wait for 30 min, at which time the pacing threshold was 2.25 V at 0.4 ms and impedance dropped to 1520 Ω. The same report described another case in which the pacing threshold was >6.5 V and impedance was 1330 Ω, but after allowing 25 min to elapse, the capture threshold decreased to 2.0 V at 0.4 ms and impedance was measured the next day at 800 Ω [9]. In fact, thresholds continued to improve in both cases the day after implant. It has been speculated that acute injury caused by the extension of the active-fixation helix being screwed into the myocardium might cause an increase in threshold that attenuates rapidly [9]. Thus, it may not always be necessary to reposition the device during implant in order to obtain adequate thresholds; instead, it requires a perioperative waiting period.

As with other implanted devices, operator experience may help reduce adverse events at implant. In an analysis of all patients implanted with a leadless pacemaker (Nanostim™) in the LEADLESS and LEADLESS II clinical trials (n = 1439), 6.4% of patients experienced a serious adverse device effect (SADE) in the first 30 days after implant, but SADE rates dropped significantly from 7.4 to 4.5% (p = 0.038), once the operator had more than 10 implants. Over time, the need for device repositioning likewise decreased with operator experience, from the first quartile (26.8%) to the fourth quartile (14.8%), p < 0.001 [10]. This suggests that there is a learning curve for leadless pacemaker implantation, not unlike that for other implantable devices, such as cardiac resynchronization therapy systems and subcutaneous implantable cardioverter defibrillators. The most frequently reported adverse events were cardiac perforation (24 events, 1.7% of patients) followed by device dislodgement (20 events, 1.4%) and tamponade (18 events, 1.3%) [10].

The leadless pacemaker is shipped already programmed to VVI pacing. It is sometimes helpful to switch the device to VOO during implant, for example, to better manage a pacemaker-dependent patient or if electromagnetic devices used during implant could potentially interfere with the pacemaker. A conventional transvenous pacemaker can be set to VOO mode perioperatively with simple magnet application, but this is not possible with some leadless pacemakers. Instead, the manufacturer or other expert team should be consulted in the event that the leadless pacemaker must be implanted in VOO mode [11].

Implant success rates are high with leadless devices. In the LEADLESS study (Nanostim™), the pacemaker could be implanted successfully in 95.8% of patients with a procedural time of 28.6 ± 17.8 min and fluoroscopy time of 13.9 ± 9.1 min [3]. In a study at a Polish single center, 10 patients were successfully implanted with a leadless pacemaker (Micra™), which was implanted with a mean implant duration of 82 min and mean fluoroscopy time of 3.5 min [12]. In a case series of five leadless pacemaker (Micra™) patients, the average duration of implantation procedure was 47 ± 11 min, which appeared to shorten over the series from a peak of 65 (second case) to 38 min for the last case [13]. In this case series, the mean capture threshold was 0.53 ± 0.27 V at 0.24 ms and mean R-wave was 13 ± 5.8 mV with no cases of acute dislodgement [13]. A study of 92 patients with leadless pacemakers (Micra™) at a Swiss single center found median capture thresholds at implant were 0.38 V at 0.24 ms (range 0.13–2.88 V at 0.24 ms), which remained stable throughout 1 year of follow-up [14]. In a case series of five leadless pacemaker patients (Micra™), all of the devices were successfully implanted [13]. A study of leadless pacing (Micra™) in Japan enrolled 38 patients at four sites and reported an implant success rate of 100% and the rate of freedom from major complications at 1 year was 96%. At 6 months, 98.3% had low, stable capture thresholds [15].

4. Safety and efficacy

4.1 Micra™ clinical studies

A prospective multicenter uncontrolled study enrolled 725 patients with an indication for single-chamber pacing to be implanted with a leadless pacemaker (Micra™). The primary endpoint was the percentage of patients with low, stable electrical capture thresholds at 6 months, defined as ≤2.0 V at 0.24 ms that increased ≤1.5 V from implant. The device could be successfully implanted in 719/725 patients (99.2%), and 96.0% met the primary endpoint at 6 months. At 6 months, the mean capture threshold was 0.54 V at 0.24 ms with an R-wave of 15.3 mV and 627 Ω impedance. The majority of patients (91%) had a pacing output of <1.5 V at 0.24 ms at 6 months, which implies that battery longevity should exceed 12 years [16]. A total of 28 major complications were reported in 25/725 patients, but no devices dislodged. Those complications included cardiac injuries (n = 11), complications at the puncture site in the groin (n = 5), thromboembolism (n = 2), pacing problems (n = 2), and other complications (n = 8). In total, three patients required device revision (two had elevated capture thresholds and one had pacemaker syndrome) and devices were deactivated (OOO mode) and abandoned; a transvenous pacing system was implanted. One patient had the device explanted because of transient loss of capture and a new leadless pacemaker was implanted [16].

A worldwide postapproval registry of the Micra™ device reported 99.1% rate of successful implantations in 1817 patients with a one-year major complication rate of 2.7% (95% confidence interval [CI], 2.0–3.7%), 63% lower than the rate of major complications for transvenous pacemaker patients (hazard ratio 0.37, 95% CI, 0.27–0.52, $p < 0.001$). In this study, there were three instances of device infection, none of which required device extraction [17].

A single-center registry of 66 patients undergoing leadless pacemaker implantation (Micra™) reported that the indications in this population were third-degree atrioventricular block, sinus node dysfunction, or permanent atrial fibrillation with bradycardia (30.3, 21.2, and 45.5%, respectively). Implant success was achieved in 65/66 patients, and electrical measurements were stable over the follow-up period of 10.4 ± 6.1 months. At the last follow-up, the mean capture threshold was 0.57 ± 0.32 V, the mean R-wave was measured at 10.62 ± 4.36 mV, and the mean impedance was 580 ± 103 Ω. In this study, one patient experienced a major adverse event (loss of device function) and there were three minor adverse events [18].

A single-arm observational study based on a postapproval registry of Micra™ leadless pacemakers reported a 99.6% success rate in device implants (792/795 patients) at 96 centers in 20 countries. At 30 days after implantation, 13 major complications were reported in 12 patients (1.51% complication rate, 95% CI, 0.78–2.62%) [19]. In a Swiss retrospective observational study of 92 Micra™ patients, the serious adverse event rate was 6.5% (n = 6), resulting in extended hospitalization for five patients and one death; three other adverse events occurred over the one-year follow-up (3.3% of patients, n = 3), resulting in revision to a conventional transvenous pacemaker in two patients and extraction of the pacemaker in the third because of ventricular tachycardia [14].

Physician acceptance of leadless pacing appears to be high. A study of leadless pacing (Micra™) in Japan enrolled 38 patients, and most of the implanting physicians said the leadless pacemaker was "extremely easy" or "easy" to implant (91.6%) and deploy (94.4%) [15].

4.2 Nanostim™ clinical trials: LEADLESS, LEADLESS II

The prospective, single-arm, multicenter LEADLESS observational study (n = 470) evaluated the freedom from serious adverse device events at 6 months as the primary endpoint. The study had to be interrupted owing to the occurrence of cardiac perforation events that required changes in the protocol and training. In the 300 patients enrolled after the study interruption, freedom from serious adverse device events was 94.6% (95% CI, 91.0–97.2%), although 18 serious adverse device events were observed in 6.6% of patients (n = 16), the most frequent of which were perforation (1.3%), vascular complications (1.3%), and dislodgement of the device (0.3%). When all 470 patients were included (before and after the interruption), 6.6% of all patients experienced a serious adverse device-related event [20].

The LEADLESS clinical trial retrospectively evaluated safety and efficacy of the Nanostim™ leadless pacemaker over a minimum of 3 years of follow-up. A total of 33 patients (mean age 77 ± 8 years) were enrolled, of whom 31 received a leadless pacemaker [21]. Two patients could not be implanted (one procedure was aborted and the other was revised to an ICD.) At 3 years, 74% (23/31) of patients were alive and no deaths were attributable to the leadless pacemaker. Most patients (89.9%) reported freedom from serious adverse events (95% CI, 79.5–100%), and 9% experienced device-related complications, of whom two had procedure-related serious adverse events. One suffered perforation leading to tamponade and the other had inadvertent implantation of the leadless pacemaker into the left ventricle by way of a patent foramen ovale, which was successfully retrieved and a new device implanted into the right ventricle. A third complication was reported after 37 months attributed to battery malfunction and necessitating device revision, which involved the successful removal of the leadless pacemaker and replacement with a new one. Up to 35 months, the electrical parameters of the leadless pacemakers were appropriate [21]. A retrospective assessment of 31 of the 33 patients from the LEADLESS study was conducted to evaluate the complication rates, device performance, and rate response features at 1 year. No pacemaker-related adverse events occurred from 3 months postimplant to 12 months. At 12 months, the mean pacing threshold was 0.43 ± 0.30 V at 0.4 ms, the mean R-wave was 10.3 ± 2.2 mV, and 61% had rate response features activated, of whom adequate results were achieved by all [22].

The LEADLESS II study is a premarket, nonrandomized, prospective, multicenter study of 526 patients with a leadless pacemaker (Nanostim™) who were followed for safety and efficacy for 6 months [3]. Inclusion criterion was a single-chamber ventricular pacing indication (which included patients with persistent or permanent atrial fibrillation). The primary efficacy outcome was achievement of a therapeutic capture threshold (defined as ≤2.0 V at 0.4 ms) and appropriate sensing (≥5.0 mV R-wave or an R-wave that exceeded the R-wave value at implant). By an intention-to-treat analysis, 90.0% of patients in the primary cohort achieved this at implant. At 12 months, the mean capture threshold was 0.58 ± 0.31 V at 0.4 ms and the mean R-wave was 9.2 ± 2.9 mV. At 12 months, the mean percentage of ventricular pacing was 51.6 ± 39.1%. The primary safety outcome was freedom from device-related adverse events in the first 6 months after implant, which was achieved by 93.3% of patients. Over 6 months, a total of 22 serious adverse events related to the device occurred in 20 patients (6.7%) in the primary cohort. In the total cohort, the rate of serious adverse events related to the device was 6.5%. Devices migrated from the heart into the pulmonary artery or right femoral vein in four and two patients, respectively, and all devices were successfully retrieved percutaneously [3]. The majority of patients did not require revision to reposition the pacemaker (70.2%), but 4.4% of patients required two or more attempts to reposition the device. The mean duration of hospital stay was 1.1 ± 1.7 days (range 0–33) [3]. Over the course of the study, 28 patients died (5.3%) but no deaths were related to the device.

The LEADLESS II patient cohort (n = 718) was compared retrospectively to 1436 transvenous pacemaker patients (historical data) with the results that leadless pacemaker patients had fewer complications (hazard ratio 0.44, 95% CI, 0.23–0.60, p < 0.001) broken down as short-term complications (5.8 vs. 9.4%, p = 0.01) and mid-term complications (0.56 vs. 4.9%, p < 0.001). Specifically, leadless pacemaker patients had more pericardial effusions (1.53 vs. 0.35%, p = 0.005), but similar rates of vascular events (1.11 vs. 0.42%, p = 0.085), dislodgements (0.97 vs. 1.39%, p = 0.54), and generator complications (0.70 vs. 0.28%, p = 0.17). Leadless pacemaker patients had no cases of thoracic trauma compared to 3.27% of transvenous patients [23].

In October 2016, an advisory was issued for the Nanostim™ device regarding premature battery depletion [24]. A prospective, observational, single-center study was conducted in Germany with patients implanted early (up until April 2014) or late (starting December 2015 and thereafter). The cohort included 14 consecutive patients (77 ± 9 years, 57% male) with a mean follow-up of 29.5 ± 11.5 months (range 11.9–44.6 months). Most were "early" patients (n = 9, 64%) implanted before the implantation suspension and five were implanted "late" (36%). From data obtained at the last follow-up, 57% had permanent atrial fibrillation with complete heart block, 21% were considered pacemaker dependent, and 36% had a mean regular escape rhythm of 37 ± 2 beats per minute (bpm). Almost half of the patients had signs of battery malfunction (43%, n = 6), all of whom had "early" implants. Using the Kaplan-Meier method, the mean time calculated from implant to device failure was 39.0 months (standard error 1.85 months, 95% CI, 35.4–42.7 months). Device parameters fell within the normal range for all patients (100%) at the last follow-up before battery malfunction was detected. Devices were explanted and analysis showed reduced electrolytes in the lithium carbon monofluoride battery, which caused high internal battery resistance, reducing the available current for device function. While a report from 2016 showed Nanostim™ battery malfunction occurred at a global rate of 2.4%, the rate at this particular institution was much higher, possibly owing to the fact that the observation period was longer [24].

4.3 Meta-analyses and comparative studies

In a meta-analysis of lead and device dislodgement (n = 18 studies, 17,321 patients) involving conventional transvenous pacemakers and leadless pacemakers (both Micra™ and Nanostim™), the weighted mean incidence of lead dislodgement in transvenous devices was 1.71%. Atrial leads had a higher dislodgement rate than ventricular leads (odds ratio 3.56, 95% CI, 1.96–6.70). The dislodgement rate for leadless devices was reported in three studies (n = 2116) and was 0, 0.13, and 1.0%, respectively, showing an overall lower dislodgement rate than conventional systems [25].

In a propensity score-matched study, 440 pacemaker patients were matched based on whether they had a leadless system (n = 220) or a transvenous system (n = 220). The complication rate at 800 days of follow-up was significantly lower in the leadless pacemaker group (0.9 vs. 4.7%, 95% CI, p = 0.02) [26].

4.4 Other safety issues

Ventricular arrhythmias after the implantation of a leadless pacemaker should be considered as potential side effect secondary to leadless pacemaker implantation. A case report in the literature describes a patient who experienced short episodes of polymorphic ventricular tachycardia (VT) in the perioperative period and high ventricular rates with short-long-short runs of polymorphic VT induced by premature ventricular contractions. The system was extracted successfully, revised with a new device of the same type successfully implanted at a different position in the right ventricle, and the VT resolved. The pro-arrhythmic effect of the leadless pacemaker remains to be elucidated, but it may involve the irritation of the right-ventricular myocardium at the site of implantation [27].

5. Leadless pacemaker features

5.1 Rate response

Both commercially available systems offer rate response. The Micra™ device utilizes a programmable accelerometer that works on three axes. Rate response is set up based on three activity vectors. The accelerometer can be programmed following a five-minute exercise test, which should be conducted before hospital discharge and then at an in-clinic visit later. While Vector 1 can be programmed as the nominal setting, an early study in 51 patients (278 tests, 818 vector measurements) found the manual selection of a vector produced better results than opting for the default Vector 1 setting. In initial testing, Vector 1 was found to be adequate in 74.5% of patients but in in-clinic testing, Vector 1 was adequate for 64.7%, while Vector 3 was adequate in 68.6% (and Vector 2 was adequate in 51.0%) [28]. The Nanostim™ device utilizes blood temperature for its rate response [2].

In the LEADLESS clinical trial (n = 31), rate response was turned on in 61% of patients at 12 months, 42% at 24 months, and 39% at 36 months [21].

5.2 Capture management

The Micra™ leadless pacemaker offers a capture management system, while the Nanostim™ does not.

5.3 Magnet mode

Application of a magnet over the implant site of a conventional transvenous pacemaker will cause it to behave in highly specific ways (for example, asynchronous fixed-rate pacing) in response in a function known as magnet mode. The Micra™ device does not offer magnet mode, but the Nanostim™ will pace at 100 bpm for eight beats and then go to asynchronous pacing at 90 bpm (or 65 bpm if the device is at the elective replacement indicator) [5].

5.4 Magnetic resonance imaging compatibility

The MIMICRY study (Monocenter Investigation Micra™ MRI Study) examined magnetic resonance imaging (MRI) compatibility in 15 leadless pacemaker patients undergoing either a 1.5 Tesla (T) or 3.0 T cardiac MRI scan; one patient was excluded from the study because severe claustrophobia precluded an MRI. Device parameters remained stable during the MRI and over the one and three-month observation points nothing showed MRI scans were safe and feasible [29]. In an *ex vivo* study using porcine hearts, leadless pacemakers were implanted in the heart (100% success rate) and then MRI conducted to assess artifacts. In most of the MRI sequences, the right ventricle and septal area near the device showed some degree of artifact, which might compromise utility, but the rest of the myocardium was free of artifacts. The leadless-pacemaker-created artifact had the shape of a shamrock and was brighter in the 3 T scans than the 1.5 T images [30].

5.5 Compatibility with external electrical cardioversion

A case report describes an 85-year-old woman with bradycardia and atrial fibrillation who received a leadless pacemaker (Micra™) and underwent external electrical cardioversion with three shocks at 100, 200, and 360 J. The three cardioversion shocks had no observable effect on the implanted leadless pacemaker [31].

6. Device retrieval

To date, there is limited experience with normal, expected end-of-life device revision. Revision may be accomplished by retrieving the old device and implanting a new one, or by simply inactivating the exhausted device and adding a new device nearby. In theory at least, device retrieval seems preferable, in that it limits the amount of hardware in the body and might reduce long-term complications or device-device interference [32]. Successful acute and chronic device retrievals have been reported in the literature. A study on human cadaver hearts has demonstrated that it is feasible to simply implant a new leadless pacemaker without removing the old one [33]. Successful device extraction in a porcine model was reported using a single-loop retrieval snare and a superior vena cava approach [34].

In a study of Micra™ pacemaker revisions, 989 implants were analyzed and compared to 2667 control patients with a transvenous ventricular single-chamber pacemaker. The actuarial rate for device revision at 24 months following implant was 1.4% for leadless pacemakers (11 revisions in 10 patients) compared to 5.3%

in the transvenous pacemaker group (123 revisions in 117 patients), that is, 75% lower for leadless pacemakers (95% CI, 53–87%, $p < 0.001$). The main reasons for extracting a leadless device were a need for a different device therapy, pacemaker syndrome, and prosthetic valve endocarditis. No leadless pacemaker was extracted because of device dislodgement or device-related infection. In seven cases, the device was deactivated and abandoned; in three cases, the device was extracted percutaneously; and in one case, the device was removed during aortic valve surgery. Overall, 64% of deactivated leadless pacemakers were left *in situ* [35].

In a retrospective study of 40 successful retrievals of leadless pacemakers (Micra™), 73% (n = 29) consented to supplying procedural details to a research study by Afzal and colleagues. This largest retrieval study to date differentiated between "immediate retrievals" (n = 11) in which the original device was retrieved perioperatively and "delayed retrieval" (n = 18) in which the retrieval involved a new procedure at a later date. The median duration between implant and retrieval in the delayed retrieval group was 46 days (range 1–95 days). The most commonly reported reasons for leadless pacemaker retrieval were elevated pacing threshold upon tether removal (immediate retrieval) and elevated threshold, endovascular infection, or need to switch to transvenous system (delayed retrieval) [36]. The mean duration for a retrieval procedure was 63.11 ± 56 min with a mean fluoroscopy exposure of 16.7 ± 9.8 min. Retrieval was accomplished using a snaring system deployed via a delivery catheter or steerable sheath. No serious complications were reported [36].

In the LEADLESS II trial, the implantable device was retrieved successfully and without complications in seven patients at 160 ± 180 days (median 100 days, 1–413 range). Of these patients, three were implanted with a new leadless pacemaker, two were implanted with a conventional transvenous pacing system, and two patients were implanted with a cardiac resynchronization therapy (CRT) device for heart failure. In a study composed of leadless pacemaker patients who required leadless pacemaker removal from three other multicenter studies, 5/5 patients who required acute extraction (within 6 weeks of implant) and 10/11 of patients who required chronic extraction (≥6 weeks after implant) experienced successful device retrieval with no procedure-related adverse events [37].

Acute explantation of the leadless device was reported in the literature when the device migrated into the pulmonary artery a few days after implantation in a 34-year-old patient with infective endocarditis. A single-loop snare guided by a steerable sheath was used to retrieve the migrated device, and a second leadless pacemaker was successfully implanted with no further complications [38]. A case report describes a 62-year-old pacemaker patient who had a leadless pacemaker implanted (to replace an infected transvenous system) and then revised with a second leadless pacemaker because of failure to capture at maximum output settings. The procedure was conducted by implanting the new leadless pacemaker into the patient, assuring its proper function, and then extracting the original underperforming leadless device using a triple-loop snare system [39]. A single-center case series reported extraction of leadless pacemakers (Nanostim™) in three cases with 100% success rate and fluoroscopic exposure times of 12, 16, and 19 min. Each extraction was preceded by a transesophageal 3D echocardiogram to assess the device's mobility with the heart and possible endothelialization. Retrieval was carried out using the proprietary catheter system from the manufacturer [40].

A novel extraction technique using a cryoballoon steerable sheath together with a snare was reported for the successful retrieval of a leadless pacemaker (Micra™), which was securely positioned in the patient but had an unusual subacute rise in pacing threshold [41]. The pacemaker was first implanted at the right-ventricular apex, but pacing thresholds were too high there (1.63 V at 0.24 ms), so the device was repositioned to a site on the right-ventricular septum with acceptable thresholds

(0.75 V at 0.24 ms). The threshold increased unexpectedly over the next 30 min to 2.2 V at 0.24 ms with no radiographic proof of dislodgement. Using a 15 French steerable cryoballoon sheath in an introducer to the right atrium, the sheath could be navigated over the tricuspid valve and into the right ventricle. A 7 French 20 mm snare was then introduced into the steerable sheath. The retrieval loop on the leadless pacemaker was successfully snared and could be extracted along with the introducer and sheath. No blood clot or visible defect was found on the extracted device. A second leadless pacemaker was implanted at the mid-septum of the right ventricle with good electrical measurements (capture threshold 0.5 V at 0.24 ms), which remained stable over 30 minutes. At 1 month, the patient has a capture threshold of 0.62 V at 0.24 ms, an R-wave of 8.6 mV, and impedance of 600 Ω [41].

Of 1423 leadless Nanostim™ pacemakers implanted around the world, there were 34 reported cases of premature battery depletion with a 90.4% successful retrieval rate even though these were chronic implants (battery depletion occurred at 2.9 ± 0.4 years). Of the seven patients in whom retrieval was not possible, most cases were caused by an inaccessible or otherwise nonfunctional retrieval loop on the device [4].

7. Quality of life

In a study of health-related quality of life using the Short-Form 36 (SF-36) questionnaire at baseline, 3 months, and 12 months in 720 Micra™ patients, all domains improved significantly at 3 and 12 months compared to baseline values and 96% were "satisfied" or "very satisfied" with the aesthetic appearance of the system, 91% with their recovery, and 74% with their current activity level [42]. Leadless pacemakers were associated with fewer restrictions on activity than leadless pacemakers in a survey of 720 patients [42].

In a study of leadless pacemaker (Micra™) patients, some national differences emerged. In this study, 35 Japanese patients were reviewed compared to 658 similar patients outside of Japan. Fewer Japanese-only patients compared to outside-Japan patients were "very satisfied" or "satisfied" with their recovery (74.3 vs. 91.8%, $p = 0.002$), but those who reported themselves "very satisfied" or "satisfied" with the device's cosmetic appearance were similar (91.4 Japanese vs. 96.2% outside Japan). All implants in the Japanese patients were successful [15].

8. Guidelines

Leadless pacemakers are indicated for patients with symptomatic bradycardia requiring single-chamber ventricular bradycardia pacing support; persistent atrial tachyarrhythmias in such patients are not a contraindication for leadless pacing. In fact, many patients who receive a leadless pacemaker have persistent or permanent atrial fibrillation with slow ventricular response.

The role of leadless pacemakers following removal of an infected conventional transvenous pacing system is debated. Since a leadless device requires no pocket formation and has no transvenous leads, it would appear to be suitable for a revision system for appropriate patients. In a study of patients who required device replacement after a conventional pacemaker system was infected ($n = 17$), patients were implanted with a Nanostim™ ($n = 11$) or Micra™ ($n = 6$) device [43]. In six patients, the leadless pacemaker was implanted within a week or less while in 11 patients, the leadless pacemakers was implanted after at least 1 week. In all patients, there was no infection over the course of a mean follow-up of 16 ± 12 months. This patient population included seven patients with a history of recurrent device infections (mean follow-up of 20 ± 14 months). This study suggests that a leadless pacemaker may be a viable revision pacing system for selected patients who experienced device infection with a conventional pacemaker [43].

The French Working Group on Cardiac Pacing and Electrophysiology of the French Society of Cardiology has issued specific guidelines on leadless pacing [44]. Currently, the indication for leadless pacing is a patient indicated for VVIR pacing and the patient's life, as well as device service life must be taken into account as device retrieval may not always be possible. They consider that leadless devices should be implanted only in centers that also perform cardiac surgery, because of the higher incidence of tamponade, vascular complications, perforations caused by large-diameter sheaths, or other complications associated with leadless pacemakers [44].

It has been recommended that anesthesiologists familiarize themselves with all implantable device technologies, including leadless pacemakers [5]. A challenge to these devices is that interrogation software may not be readily available and that implantation should be coordinated with device manufacturer representatives or cardiologists, for example, if the device should be programmed to an asynchronous pacing mode during implant [5].

9. Special populations

In 64% of patients enrolled in one of the pivotal trials for leadless pacemakers (Micra™), the pacing indication was managing persistent or permanent atrial fibrillation with slow ventricular response [16]. In that pivotal trial, only 6% of patients had a clear-cut medical reason that limited or contraindicated them from a transvenous system. However, there are many emerging groups who may derive benefits from leadless pacemakers.

9.1 Limited or occluded venous access

Leadless pacemakers may be an important alternative to conventional devices in patients with thromboses, venous obstruction, tortuous or abnormal venous anatomy, superior vena cava syndrome, or other conditions may be contraindicated for a conventional transvenous pacemaker. A case report describes a patient with third-degree atrioventricular (AV) block who experienced an occlusive thrombosis of the superior vena cava and had her conventional VDD transvenous pacemaker replaced with a leadless device [45]. Limited venous access as an anatomical challenge may be overcome with a leadless pacemaker as in a case study of a bradycardic hemodialysis patient who suffered from skin erosion in the chest area due to radiation treatments for esophageal carcinoma. The leadless pacemaker was implanted successfully, but the patient developed ventricular tachyarrhythmias, necessitating the implantation of a subcutaneous implantable cardioverter-defibrillator. At 1 month, both devices were performing adequately with no device-device interactions [46].

A 72-year-old man with a thrombosed venous stent, renal failure, and myelodysplastic syndrome presented with second-degree AV block. A leadless pacemaker was preferred (Micra™) because of limited venous access and a high risk of infection due to his immunocompromised condition [47].

9.2 Pacemaker-dependent patients transitioned to leadless pacing

When it is necessary to extract transvenous leads in a pacemaker-dependent patient, a common approach is to utilize a temporary pacemaker with active-fixation lead as a bridge to a contralateral pacemaker implantation. A case report describes the use of a leadless pacemaker in a pacemaker-dependent patient with dextrocardia who required lead extraction following endocarditis. The implantation procedure was uneventful and the leadless pacemaker performed well with stable measurements taken 1 year postimplant [48].

9.3 Transplanted hearts

The literature reports on successful implantation of a leadless pacemaker in a transplanted heart [49].

9.4 Patients with prosthetic valves

The permanent position of a transvenous lead over the tricuspid valve may cause damage to the valve. In patients with a prosthetic tricuspid valve, locating a transvenous lead over the tricuspid valve must be considered carefully. The literature reports a case in which a 67-year-old woman with three valve replacements (an aortic mechanical valve, a mitral mechanical valve, and a tricuspid prosthesis) underwent successful implantation of a leadless pacemaker (Micra™) for high-degree AV block with permanent atrial fibrillation. She had previously had an epicardial pacemaker, which experienced lead dysfunction and transient loss of capture [50].

In a study of 23 leadless pacemaker patients (both Micra™ and Nanostim™), devices were implanted in the septal-apical area or the mid-septal region of the right ventricle. No observed changes in heart structure or heart function, such as changes to the tricuspid valve, were found. One patient in this study developed increased tricuspid valve regurgitation but without abnormal leaflet motion or any changes in annulus size, suggesting it was caused by changes in right ventricular pressure [51].

9.5 Tandem subcutaneous ICD with leadless pacemaker

It is not difficult to imagine the possibilities of combining a subcutaneous ICD (S-ICD) with a leadless pacemaker to allow for bradycardia pacing support and rescue defibrillation in a patient without the need for any transvenous leads. In an experimental study (n = 40, animal models were ovine, porcine, and canine), the dual devices were successfully implanted in 39/40 and 23 animals were followed for 90 days. Appropriate pacing was observed in 100% of animals by the leadless pacemaker, and the ICD could communicate unidirectionally with the pacemaker in 99% of cases. When triggered, the leadless pacemaker could deliver antitachycardia pacing (10 beats at 81% of the coupling interval) in 100% of attempts, while the S-ICD was able to maintain appropriate sensing [52]. While this is a preliminary animal study, it demonstrates the potential of utilizing these two leadless systems in tandem. For an S-ICD and a leadless pacemaker to work effectively together, they require the ability to communicate with each other, which, in turn, depends on the device orientation within the subject. In a canine study (n = 23), it was found that communication could occur in 100% of the implanted dogs although the median angle of the leadless pacemaker was 29°, and the median distance of the S-ICD to the leadless pacemaker was 0.8 cm. While these are not optimal values, communication was effective. A retrospective study of 72 leadless pacemaker patients found the median angle of the leadless pacemaker was 56 degrees; in a retrospective analysis of 100 S-ICD patients, the median distance between the coil and the position of the leadless pacemaker was 4.6 cm [53]. Thus, it appears that communication between devices is possible and that humans offer a better theoretical positioning opportunity for such communication than dogs.

Dual device implantation was performed in an 81-year-old man who received an S-ICD in 2012 after explant of three transvenous ICDs due to infection [54]. At the time of S-ICD implant, the patient had no indication for bradycardia pacing, but that changed in 2015 when he developed sinus bradycardia with a daytime heart rate of about 20 bpm. Both subclavian veins were occluded, and it was decided to implant a leadless pacemaker (Micra™). The device was successfully implanted with satisfactory electrical measurements (capture threshold was 0.38 V at 0.24 ms capture threshold, the R-wave was 10.4 mV, and impedance was 640 Ω). When programmed to high outputs, the leadless pacemaker did not appear to interact with the S-ICD, even at its most sensitive settings. The patient was doing well with improved function at 4 months. At 6 months, the patient had a VT that was appropriately sensed and converted at first shock. The threshold of the leadless pacemaker following the shock remained stable [54].

9.6 Dialysis patients

For patients with chronic renal disease, a leadless pacemaker may allow preservation for central veins, necessary for permanent dialysis vascular access [55]. In patients with end-stage renal disease and the need for an implantable pacemaker, it is best to avoid transvenous leads if possible. Since kidney disease can progress rapidly, patients with a high risk for renal failure (for example, glomerular filtration rate < 20 mL/min/1.73 m^2); it may be helpful to consider these patients for leadless pacemakers or S-ICD systems rather than transvenous devices when possible [56].

9.7 Patients with indwelling inferior vena cava filters

Leadless pacemakers are contraindicated in patients with an indwelling inferior vena cava (IVC) filter, but as IVC filters become more common, the role of leadless pacemakers in this population will be explored. In some cases, an IVC filter might block passage of a catheter entering the femoral vein and routing toward the heart, but there are cases reported in the literature in which the catheter with the leadless pacemaker has been able to navigate around the indwelling IVC device. However, large studies of leadless pacemakers exclude IVC filter patients, so there is not much data on how a leadless pacemaker might be deployed in this population. A few cases in the literature suggest it is feasible, at least in selected cases, to implant a leadless pacemaker in the presence of an IVC filter.

A case report in the literature describes the successful implant of a Micra™ device via a collateral branch of the right common femoral vein through a previously implanted IVC filter in a 68-year-old man with a history of pulmonary embolism and recent development of AV block [57].

9.8 Left atrial appendage occluders

There is a report in the literature of a dual implant of a left-atrial-appendage occluder (Watchman™, Boston Scientific, Natick, Massachusetts, USA) and a leadless pacemaker (Micra™) in a single procedure. The patient was a 73-year-old woman with persistent atrial fibrillation. Both devices were implanted via right femoral access with no complications and good results at 1 month postimplant [58].

9.9 Small patients

The idea that this miniaturized pacemaker might be appropriate in smaller patients has been explored in a few case studies. The literature reports a successful implantation of a leadless device (Micra™) in an 11-year-old patient with recurrent syncopal episodes and prolonged sinus pauses [59]. A 71-year-old man with achondroplastic dwarfism had a transvenous pacemaker for decades for third-degree AV block; in 2010, a pocket infection with endocarditis of the tricuspid valve necessitated the extraction of the conventional pacemaker and placement of an epicardial dual-chamber pacemaker with tunneling of leads. The patient was pacemaker dependent with permanent atrial fibrillation and developed an untreatable pocket infection. He was implanted with a leadless pacemaker (Micra™) via standard implantation technique, which was complicated by the fact that the delivery catheter was much longer than the patient's inferior limb. The device was successfully implanted and showed good electrical results. The epicardial device was then removed via a mini-thoracotomy [60]. A leadless pacemaker (Micra™) could be successfully implanted in a small-frame geriatric patient with third-degree AV block and a history of pacemaker implantations and infections [61].

9.10 Vasovagal syncope

A leadless pacemaker was successfully implanted in a 17-year-old male patient with cardioinhibitory syncope. The patient had vasovagal syncope with episodes of bradycardia and drops in arterial blood pressure. An implantable loop recorder documented a pause of 9 s, whereupon he was implanted with the leadless pacemaker [62]. Cardioinhibitory syncope may be a temporary condition.

9.11 AV nodal ablation with permanent pacing

For rate control in patients with symptomatic atrial fibrillation (AF), atrioventricular (AV) nodal ablation with subsequent pacemaker implantation (the so-called "ablate and pace" procedure) is an established course of treatment. In a multicenter observational study of 127 such patients, 60 received a leadless pacemaker and 67 a conventional transvenous pacemaker. The primary efficacy endpoint of this study was acceptable sensing thresholds (R wave ≥ 5.0 mV and pacing threshold ≤ 2.0 V at 0.4 ms). Nearly all patients (95% in leadless and 97% in conventional groups) met the primary endpoint. Five early and one late minor adverse events occurred in the leadless pacemaker group and three early adverse events occurred in the conventional pacemaker group (not statistically significantly different). Thus, it appears that leadless pacemakers may be a viable option for "ablate and pace" patients [63]. In another study in a similar population, 21 patients with permanent atrial fibrillation underwent implantation of a leadless pacemaker (Micra™) followed by AV junctional ablation; these patients were followed over 12 months with no major device-related complications. Two patients in this study died over the course of the 12 month follow-up of noncardiac causes [64]. Short- and long-term outcomes of patients undergoing a simultaneous leadless pacemaker implantation were reported from an observational study of 137 patients (mean age 77.9 ± 10.5 years) in which 19.7% (n = 37) underwent simultaneous AV nodal ablation. The complication rate was 5.5% in patients who just had leadless pacemaker insertion and 11% in those who underwent both ablation and pacemaker implant. There were no cases of device dislodgement in either group. Over the mean follow-up of 123 ± 48 days, 3.6% patients (n = 3) died, but all deaths were unrelated to cardiovascular causes. There were no significant differences between groups in terms of pacing and sensing threshold values [65].

9.12 Concurrent valve replacement and pacemaker implantation

The literature reports on a 66-year-old female with rheumatic heart disease, permanent atrial fibrillation with slow ventricular response, and renal failure. She was admitted for mitral valve replacement and tricuspid valve repair, at which time a *de novo* pacemaker would be implanted to help manage transient AV block. It was decided to implant a leadless pacemaker (Micra™), but the sequence of these three procedures (valve replacement, valve repair, and pacemaker implantation) was not clear. The device was anchored at an adjacent septal site with measurements of 1.25 V at 0.24 ms capture threshold, R-wave of 7 mV, and impedance of 600 Ω. After this satisfactory implantation was achieved, a tricuspid ring annuloplasty was carried out successfully, and the proper position of the leadless pacemaker was confirmed using intraoperative transesophageal echocardiography [66].

The literature reports a case in which a 91-year-old man underwent a successful transcatheter aortic valve implantation (TAVI) but experienced the not uncommon side effect of conduction disturbances. As the patient was frail and elderly, it was decided to implant a leadless pacemaker to help manage the arrhythmias rather than a transvenous system. The procedure was successful and the patient was discharged without complications [67].

9.13 Congenital heart disorders

Patients with congenital heart disorders are at an elevated risk for arrhythmias and anatomical anomalies, which may complicate venous access and device implantation. In fact, congenital heart disease patients have a rate for pacemaker-related complications that approaches 40% compared to about 5% in the general population [68]. A case study in the literature reports on a 47-year-old female pacemaker-dependent patient with congenital heart disease who had experienced complications with a transvenous pacemaker (lead malfunction followed by occlusion of the superior vena cava and innominate veins). The transvenous lead was abandoned, and the patient was revised to an epicardial system. She presented with dizzy spells, and it was found her epicardial system was nearing end of service and had elevated thresholds. As there was no viable vascular access, it was decided to revise her pacemaker to a leadless system (Micra™). The leadless pacemaker was implanted via left femoral venous access and a steerable catheter to the right ventricular apical septal region where it was successfully positioned with good electrical values (1.0 V at 0.4 ms with an R-wave of 8 mV) [69].

10. Costs

At present, leadless pacemakers cost significantly more than a conventional transvenous device without the expense of two transvenous leads. The question of cost effectiveness in medical devices is always complicated, but it must be taken into account that even with a higher upfront cost, leadless pacemakers have substantially longer expected longevity (up to twice as long as a conventional transvenous pacemaker) and fewer complications [13]. In an online survey conducted by the European Heart Rhythm Association (EHRA) of 52 centers who participate in the EHRA Research Network, most of the 52 centers who reported said they implanted leadless pacemakers (86%) but at a small volume (82% said they implanted fewer than 30 such devices in the past 12 months). The main reasons for the low volume were device costs (91%) and lack of reimbursement for these systems (55%) [50].

11. Future challenges

Currently, leadless pacing is limited to right-ventricular pacing only. The vast majority of pacemaker patients depend on AV synchronization and may even benefit from additional cardiac resynchronization for heart failure. One way to solve the AV-sequential issue is to employ VDD mode that would allow for atrial sensing; a subcutaneous ECG integrated into the circuit would be an option.

Systems that are able to communicate between devices are being developed, i.e., integration of a leadless pacemaker with an S-ICD. Ideally, this combination would offer reliable sensing/pacing in the right ventricle including antitachycardia pacing in order to terminate VT without shock therapy. Moreover, combining intracardiac signals from the leadless pacemaker with the subcutaneous ECG from the S-ICD may improve the system's ability to discriminate arrhythmias.

Another concern is handling of the device at the end of its service life. Likely, the devices will be encapsulated and could be programmed off (OOO mode), and up to three devices can reasonably be accommodated within the right ventricle [33]. However, many pacemaker patients are old with a shorter life expectancy than projected batter longevity and will only need one device.

Extraction will be necessary in the event of an infection, and the development of safe catheter-based tools would be helpful even in the situation of complete device encapsulation. More data are needed about safety of leadless pacemakers with regard to infection, device migration, and RV failure in long-term follow-up.

A leadless ultrasound-based technology used by the WiCS™ system (Wireless Cardiac Stimulation, EBR Systems) has been developed for endocardial pacing of the left ventricle [70]. The ultrasound energy is transmitted from a subcutaneous transmitter to an endocardial receiver unit in the endocardium. This device is fixed by three self-expanding nitinol tines on the device. Thus, this cardiac resynchronization therapy (CRT) system comprises three parts: the left-ventricular endocardial unit (using ultrasound for conversion of electrical energy), the subcutaneous pulse generator, and a conventional pacing device. The subcutaneously implanted pulse generator consists of a battery connected by a cable to a transmitter. The system detects right-ventricular stimulation provided by the concomitant pacemaker, CRT device, or ICD.

12. Conclusion

The technology of leadless pacing is a disruptive innovation with the potential to usher in a new era of cardiac pacing and solve problems related to the transvenous leads and pocket. The first-generation leadless pacemakers are limited to single-chamber pacing, typically VVIR pacing, but further innovations may expand that. Battery longevity is supposed to be excellent, but real-world clinical data are needed from long-term use to confirm this. The extraction of a leadless pacemaker remains a challenge. Future directions include integration of leadless pacing with S-ICDs, dual-chamber devices, and a leadless version of CRT pacing.

Acknowledgements

Todd Cooper of Coyote Studios in Los Angeles, California, provided the original illustration. The authors acknowledge editorial assistance provided by John Bisney who proofed the final manuscript. Trademarks and registered trademarks in this chapter are the property of their respective owners.

Conflict of interest

The authors have no relevant conflicts to disclose.

Author details

Peter Magnusson[1,2], Joseph V. Pergolizzi Jr [3] and Jo Ann LeQuang[3]*

1 Cardiology Research Unit, Department of Medicine, Karolinska Institute, Stockholm, Sweden

2 Centre for Research and Development, Uppsala University/Region Gävleborg, Gävle, Sweden

3 NEMA Research, Inc., Naples, Florida, USA

*Address all correspondence to: joann@leqmedical.com

References

[1] Cano Perez O, Pombo Jimenez M, Fidalgo Andres ML, Lorente Carreno D, Coma Samartin R. Spanish Pacemaker Registry. 14th Official Report of the Spanish Society of Cardiology Working Group on Cardiac Pacing (2016). Revista Espanola de Cardiologia (English ed). 2017;**70**(12):1083-1097

[2] Kancharla K, Deshmukh AJ, Friedman PA. Leadless pacemakers—Implant, explant and long-term safety and efficacy data. Journal of Atrial Fibrillation. 2017;**10**(2):1581

[3] Reddy VY, Exner DV, Cantillon DJ, Doshi R, Bunch TJ, Tomassoni GF, et al. Percutaneous implantation of an entirely intracardiac leadless pacemaker. The New England Journal of Medicine. 2015;**373**(12):1125-1135

[4] Lakkireddy D, Knops R, Atwater B, Neuzil P, Ip J, Gonzalez E, et al. A worldwide experience of the management of battery failures and chronic device retrieval of the Nanostim leadless pacemaker. Heart Rhythm: The Official Journal of the Heart Rhythm Society. 2017;**14**(12):1756-1763

[5] Cronin B, Essandoh MK. Update on cardiovascular implantable electronic devices for anesthesiologists. Journal of Cardiothoracic and Vascular Anesthesia. 2018;**32**(4):1871-1884

[6] Kolek MJ, Crossley GH, Ellis CR. Implantation of a MICRA leadless pacemaker via right internal jugular vein. JACC Clinical Electrophysiology. 2018;**4**(3):420-421

[7] Lloyd MS, El-Chami MF, Nilsson KR Jr, Cantillon DJ. Transcatheter/leadless pacing. Heart Rhythm: The Official Journal of the Heart Rhythm Society. 2018;**15**(4):624-628

[8] Conyers JM, Rajiah P, Ahn R, Abbara S, Saboo SS. Imaging features of leadless cardiovascular devices. Diagnostic and Interventional Radiology (Ankara, Turkey). 2018;**24**(4):203-208

[9] Kawata H, Patel PM, Banker R. Nanostim leadless pacemaker system: A longer waiting period after active fixation may reduce unnecessary repositioning. HeartRhythm Case Reports. 2018;**4**(2):63-65

[10] Tjong FVY, Beurskens NEG, Neuzil P, Defaye P, Delnoy PP, Ip J, et al. The learning curve associated with the implantation of the Nanostim leadless pacemaker. Journal of Interventional Cardiac Electrophysiology: An International Journal of Arrhythmias and Pacing. 2018;**53**(2):239-247

[11] Essandoh M. Perioperative management of the micra leadless pacemaker. Journal of Cardiothoracic and Vascular Anesthesia. 2017;**31**(6):e97-ee8

[12] Grabowski M, Michalak M, Gawalko M, Gajda S, Cacko A, Januszkiewicz L, et al. Implantation of the Micra transcatheter pacing system: Single Polish center experience with the real costs of hospitalization analysis. Cardiology Journal. 2018

[13] Shen EN, Ishihara CH, Uehara DR. Leadless pacemaker: Report of the first experience in Hawai'i. Hawai'i Journal of Medicine & Public Health: A Journal of Asia Pacific Medicine & Public Health. 2018;**77**(4):79-82

[14] Valiton V, Graf D, Pruvot E, Carroz P, Fromer M, Bisch L, et al. Leadless pacing using the transcatheter pacing system (Micra TPS) in the real world: Initial Swiss experience from the Romandie region. Europace. 2018

[15] Soejima K, Asano T, Ishikawa T, Kusano K, Sato T, Okamura H, et al. Performance of leadless pacemaker in

japanese patients vs. rest of the world—Results from a global clinical trial. Circulation Journal: Official Journal of the Japanese Circulation Society. 2017;**81**(11):1589-1595

[16] Reynolds D, Duray GZ, Omar R, Soejima K, Neuzil P, Zhang S, et al. A leadless intracardiac transcatheter pacing system. The New England Journal of Medicine. 2016;**374**(6):533-541

[17] El-Chami MF, Al-Samadi F, Clementy N, Garweg C, Martinez-Sande JL, Piccini JP, et al. Updated performance of the Micra transcatheter pacemaker in the real-world setting: A comparison to the investigational study and a transvenous historical control. Heart Rhythm: The Official Journal of the Heart Rhythm Society. 2018

[18] Garweg C, Ector J, Voros G, Greyling A, Vandenberk B, Foulon S, et al. Monocentric experience of leadless pacing with focus on challenging cases for conventional pacemaker. Acta Cardiologica. 2018;**73**(5):459-468

[19] Roberts PR, Clementy N, Al Samadi F, Garweg C, Martinez-Sande JL, Iacopino S, et al. A leadless pacemaker in the real-world setting: The Micra Transcatheter Pacing System Post-Approval Registry. Heart Rhythm: The Official Journal of the Heart Rhythm Society. 2017;**14**(9):1375-1379

[20] Sperzel J, Defaye P, Delnoy PP, Garcia Guerrero JJ, Knops RE, Tondo C, et al. Primary safety results from the LEADLESS Observational Study. Europace. 2018

[21] Tjong FVY, Knops RE, Neuzil P, Petru J, Sediva L, Wilde AAM, et al. Midterm safety and performance of a leadless cardiac pacemaker: 3-year follow-up to the LEADLESS Trial (Nanostim Safety and Performance Trial for a Leadless Cardiac Pacemaker System). Circulation. 2018;**137**(6):633-635

[22] Knops RE, Tjong FV, Neuzil P, Sperzel J, Miller MA, Petru J, et al. Chronic performance of a leadless cardiac pacemaker: 1-year follow-up of the LEADLESS trial. Journal of the American College of Cardiology. 2015;**65**(15):1497-1504

[23] Cantillon DJ, Dukkipati SR, Ip JH, Exner DV, Niazi IK, Banker RS, et al. Comparative study of acute and mid-term complications with leadless and transvenous cardiac pacemakers. Heart Rhythm: The Official Journal of the Heart Rhythm Society. 2018;**15**(7):1023-1030

[24] Richter S, Doring M, Ebert M, Bode K, Mussigbrodt A, Sommer P, et al. Battery malfunction of a leadless cardiac pacemaker: Worrisome single-center experience. Circulation. 2018;**137**(22):2408-2410

[25] Wang Y, Hou W, Zhou C, Yin Y, Lu S, Liu G, et al. Meta-analysis of the incidence of lead dislodgement with conventional and leadless pacemaker systems. Pacing and Clinical Electrophysiology: PACE. 2018

[26] Tjong FVY, Knops RE, Udo EO, Brouwer TF, Dukkipati SR, Koruth JS, et al. Leadless pacemaker versus transvenous single-chamber pacemaker therapy: A propensity score-matched analysis. Heart Rhythm: The Official Journal of the Heart Rhythm Society. 2018;**15**(9):1387-1393

[27] Amin AK, Billakanty SR, Chopra N, Fu EY, Nichols AJ, Kleman JM, et al. Premature ventricular contraction-induced polymorphic ventricular tachycardia after leadless pacemaker implantation: A unique adverse effect of leadless pacing. HeartRhythm Case Reports. 2018;**4**(5):180-183

[28] Bari Z, Vamos M, Bogyi P, Reynolds D, Sheldon T, Fagan DH, et al. Physical activity detection in patients with intracardiac leadless pacemaker. Journal

of Cardiovascular Electrophysiology. 2018

[29] Blessberger H, Kiblboeck D, Reiter C, Lambert T, Kellermair J, Schmit P, et al. Monocenter Investigation Micra(R) MRI study (MIMICRY): Feasibility study of the magnetic resonance imaging compatibility of a leadless pacemaker system. Europace. 2018

[30] Edlinger C, Granitz M, Paar V, Jung C, Pfeil A, Eder S, et al. Visualization and appearance of artifacts of leadless pacemaker systems in cardiac MRI : An experimental ex vivo study. Wiener Klinische Wochenschrift. 2018;**130**(13-14):427-435

[31] Filipovic K, Bellmann B, Luker J, Steven D, Sultan A. External electrical cardioversion of persistent atrial fibrillation in a patient with a Micra Transcatheter Pacing System. Indian Pacing and Electrophysiology Journal. 2018;**18**(1):44-46

[32] Beurskens NE, Tjong FV, Knops RE. End-of-life management of leadless cardiac pacemaker therapy. Arrhythmia & Electrophysiology Review. 2017;**6**(3):129-133

[33] Omdahl P, Eggen MD, Bonner MD, Iaizzo PA, Wika K. Right ventricular anatomy can accommodate multiple micra transcatheter pacemakers. Pacing and Clinical Electrophysiology: PACE. 2016;**39**(4):393-397

[34] Vatterott PJ, Eggen MD, Mattson AR, Omdahl PK, Hilpisch KE, Iaizzo PA. Retrieval of a chronically implanted leadless pacemaker within an isolated heart using direct visualization. HeartRhythm Case Reports. 2018;**4**(5):167-169

[35] Grubman E, Ritter P, Ellis CR, Giocondo M, Augostini R, Neuzil P, et al. To retrieve, or not to retrieve: System revisions with the Micra transcatheter pacemaker. Heart Rhythm: The Official Journal of the Heart Rhythm Society. 2017;**14**(12):1801-1806

[36] Afzal MR, Daoud EG, Cunnane R, Mulpuru SK, Koay A, Hussain A, et al. Techniques for successful early retrieval of the Micra transcatheter pacing system: A worldwide experience. Heart Rhythm: The Official Journal of the Heart Rhythm Society. 2018;**15**(6):841-846

[37] Reddy VY, Miller MA, Knops RE, Neuzil P, Defaye P, Jung W, et al. Retrieval of the leadless cardiac pacemaker: A multicenter experience. Circulation. Arrhythmia and Electrophysiology. 2016;**9**(12):pii:e004626

[38] Taborsky M, Skala T, Kocher M, Fedorco M. Extraction of a dislocated leadless pacemaker in a patient with infective endocarditis and repeated endocardial and epicardial pacing system infections. Biomedical Papers of the Medical Faculty of the University Palacky, Olomouc, Czechoslovakia. 2018

[39] M RA, Dar T, Houmsse M, Augostini R, Daoud EG, Hummel J. Successful denovo implantation and explanation of an old malfunctioning micratm leadless pacemaker. Journal of Atrial Fibrillation. 2017;**10**(4):1723

[40] Gonzalez Villegas E, Al Razzo O, Silvestre Garcia J, Mesa Garcia J. Leadless pacemaker extraction from a single-center perspective. Pacing and Clinical Electrophysiology: PACE. 2018;**41**(2):101-105

[41] Chan NY, Yuen HC, Mok NS. Successful percutaneous retrieval of a leadless pacemaker due to an acute rise in pacing threshold. Indian Pacing and Electrophysiology Journal. 2017;**17**(6):186-188

[42] Tjong FVY, Beurskens NEG, de Groot JR, Waweru C, Liu S, Ritter P,

et al. Health-related quality of life impact of a transcatheter pacing system. Journal of Cardiovascular Electrophysiology. 2018

[43] Beurskens NEG, Tjong FVY, Dasselaar KJ, Kuijt WJ, Wilde AAM, Knops RE. Leadless pacemaker implantation after explantation of infected conventional pacemaker systems: A viable solution? Heart Rhythm: The Official Journal of the Heart Rhythm Society. 2018

[44] Defaye P, Klug D, Anselme F, Gras D, Hermida JS, Piot O, et al. Recommendations for the implantation of leadless pacemakers from the French Working Group on Cardiac Pacing and Electrophysiology of the French Society of Cardiology. Archives of Cardiovascular Diseases. 2018;**111**(1):53-58

[45] Dell'Era G, Porcellini S, Boggio E, Prenna E, Gravellone M, Varalda M, et al. Transcatheter leadless pacemaker implantation in a patient with failing transvenous pacemaker and total occlusion of superior vena cava. Journal of Cardiovascular Medicine (Hagerstown, Md). 2018;**19**(9):511-512

[46] Enomoto Y, Hashimoto H, Ishii R, Torii S, Nakamura K, Noro M, et al. Leadless pacemaker and subcutaneous implantable cardioverter defibrillator combination in a hemodialysis patient. Circulation Journal: Official Journal of the Japanese Circulation Society. 2018

[47] Sideris S, Archontakis S, Vaina S, Stroumpouli E, Koumallos N, Gatzoulis K, et al. Leadless pacing systems: A valuable alternative for patients with severe access problems. Hellenic Journal of Cardiology: HJC = Hellenike kardiologike epitheorese. 2018;**59**(1):36-39

[48] De Regibus V, Pardeo A, Artale P, Petretta A, Filannino P, Iacopino S. Leadless pacemaker implantation after transcatheter lead extraction in complex anatomy patient. Clinical Case Reports. 2018;**6**(6):1106-1108

[49] Martinez-Sande JL, Garcia-Seara J, Gonzalez-Melchor L, Rodriguez-Manero M, Gomez-Otero I, Gonzalez-Juanatey JR. Leadless pacemaker implantation in a transplanted heart. Revista Espanola de Cardiologia (English ed). 2018

[50] Boveda S, Lenarczyk R, Haugaa KH, Iliodromitis K, Finlay M, Lane D, et al. Use of leadless pacemakers in Europe: Results of the European Heart Rhythm Association survey. Europace. 2018;**20**(3):555-559

[51] Salaun E, Tovmassian L, Simonnet B, Giorgi R, Franceschi F, Koutbi-Franceschi L, et al. Right ventricular and tricuspid valve function in patients chronically implanted with leadless pacemakers. Europace. 2018;**20**(5):823-828

[52] Tjong FVY, Brouwer TF, Koop B, Soltis B, Shuros A, Schmidt B, et al. Acute and 3-month performance of a communicating leadless antitachycardia pacemaker and subcutaneous implantable defibrillator. JACC Clinical Electrophysiology. 2017;**3**(13):1487-1498

[53] Quast ABE, Tjong FVY, Koop BE, Wilde AAM, Knops RE, Burke MC. Device orientation of a leadless pacemaker and subcutaneous implantable cardioverter-defibrillator in canine and human subjects and the effect on intrabody communication. Europace. 2018

[54] Ahmed FZ, Cunnington C, Motwani M, Zaidi AM. Totally leadless dual-device implantation for combined spontaneous ventricular tachycardia defibrillation and pacemaker function: A first report. The Canadian Journal of Cardiology. 2017;**33**(8):1066.e5-1066.e7

[55] Maradey JA, Jao GT, Vachharajani TJ. Leadless pacemaker placement

in a patient with chronic kidney disease: A strategy to preserve central veins. Hemodialysis International International Symposium on Home Hemodialysis. 2018

[56] Kusztal M, Nowak K. Cardiac implantable electronic device and vascular access: Strategies to overcome problems. The Journal of Vascular Access. 2018:1129729818762981

[57] Flores E, Patel M, Orme G, Su W. Successful implantation of a Micra leadless pacemaker via collateral femoral vein and inferior vena cava filter. Clinical Case Reports. 2018;**6**(3):502-505

[58] Johar S, Luqman N. Implant of a left atrial appendage occluder device (Watchman) and leadless pacing system (Micra) through the same venous access in a single sitting. BMJ Case Reports. 2018;**2018**

[59] Tejman-Yarden S, Nof E, Beinart R, Ovadia N, Goldshmit Y, Buber J, et al. Leadless pacemaker implantation in a pediatric patient with prolonged sinus pauses. Pediatric Cardiology. 2018;**39**(4):844-847

[60] Morani G, Bolzan B, Borio G, Tomasi L, Ribichini FL. Leadless pacemaker implantation in achondroplastic dwarfism and recurrent cardiac implantable electronic device infections: A case report. Europace. 2018;**20**(7):1160

[61] Tse G, Liu T, Li G, Tak Wong W, Chin Pang Chan G, Chan YS, et al. Implantation of the Micra leadless pacemaker in a patient with a low body mass index of 16. Oxford Medical Case Reports. 2017;**2017**(9):omx051

[62] De Regibus V, Moran D, Chierchia GB, Brugada P, de Asmundis C. Leadless pacing in a young patient with cardioinhibitory vasovagal syncope. Indian Pacing and Electrophysiology Journal. 2018;**18**(3):120-122

[63] Yarlagadda B, Turagam MK, Dar T, Janagam P, Veerapaneni V, Atkins D, et al. Safety and feasibility of leadless pacemaker in patients undergoing atrioventricular node ablation for atrial fibrillation. Heart Rhythm: The Official Journal of the Heart Rhythm Society. 2018;**15**(7):994-1000

[64] Okabe T, El-Chami MF, Lloyd MS, Buck B, Gornick CC, Moore JC, et al. Leadless pacemaker implantation and concurrent atrioventricular junction ablation in patients with atrial fibrillation. Pacing and Clinical Electrophysiology: PACE. 2018;**41**(5):504-510

[65] Martinez-Sande JL, Rodriguez-Manero M, Garcia-Seara J, Lago M, Gonzalez-Melchor L, Kreidieh B, et al. Acute and long-term outcomes of simultaneous atrioventricular node ablation and leadless pacemaker implantation. Pacing and Clinical Electrophysiology: PACE. 2018

[66] Marai I, Diab S, Ben-Avi R, Kachel E. Intraoperative implantation of micra leadless pacemaker during valve surgery. The Annals of Thoracic Surgery. 2018;**105**(5):e211-e2e2

[67] Shikama T, Miura M, Shirai S, Hayashi M, Morita J, Nagashima M, et al. Leadless pacemaker implantation following transcatheter aortic valve implantation using SAPIEN 3. Korean Circulation Journal. 2018;**48**(6):534-535

[68] McLeod CJ, Attenhofer Jost CH, Warnes CA, Hodge D 2nd, Hyberger L, Connolly HM, et al. Epicardial versus endocardial permanent pacing in adults with congenital heart disease. Journal of Interventional Cardiac Electrophysiology: An International Journal of Arrhythmias and Pacing. 2010;**28**(3):235-243

[69] Sanhoury M, Fassini G, Tundo F, Moltrasio M, Ribatti V, Lumia G, et al. Rescue leadless pacemaker implantation

in a pacemaker-dependent patient with congenital heart disease and no alternative routes for pacing. Journal of Atrial Fibrillation. 2017;**9**(5):1542

[70] Sperzel J, Burri H, Gras D, Tjong FV, Knops RE, Hindricks G, et al. State of the art of leadless pacing. Europace. 2015;**17**(10):1508-1513

Chapter 5

Atrial Fibrillation and the Role of Thumb ECGs

Peter Magnusson, Magnus Samuelsson, Joseph V. Pergolizzi Jr, Hani Annabi and Jo Ann LeQuang

Abstract

Atrial fibrillation (AF) may be underdiagnosed, and there is much that remains unknown about this prevalent and potentially life-threatening arrhythmia. AF epidemiology has been thwarted in part by the fact that about a third of patients with AF have no symptoms, those with symptoms may experience them intermittently or have vague symptoms, and it can be challenging to capture an episode on a 12-lead ECG, which is required for diagnosis. There are many significant knowledge gaps in our understanding of AF etiology and progression. A new user-friendly device that allows for frequent self-monitoring of the heart rhythm has been introduced. With the thumb ECG, patients can record a tracing multiple times a day. A smartphone app will soon allow them to interact with their healthcare providers about these ECG recordings. An ECG parser will allow for an algorithm-directed, rapid, automatic interpretation of these recordings with high specificity and sensitivity. This may help researchers learn more about the so-called *silent AF,* AF progression (and possible remission), and risk factors for AF. This technology holds great promise for patient care as well as for research into AF.

Keywords: arrhythmia, atrial fibrillation, thumb ECG, Coala heart monitor, stroke

1. Introduction

Atrial fibrillation (AF) is the most common sustained arrhythmia and associated with a fivefold increased risk of stroke and a threefold increased risk of heart failure; thus, AF is a major cause of cardiovascular morbidity [1–3]. The European Society of Cardiology (ESC) recognizes five main types of AF: first diagnosed episode, paroxysmal, persistent, long-standing persistent, and permanent [3] (see **Table 1**). It had long been thought that *AF begets AF* and the arrhythmia followed a linear forward progression from short, infrequent, self-terminating episodes to more persistent forms of AF, but that paradigm has been challenged in that about 3% of patients seem to have paroxysmal AF that never advances to more persistent forms [4]. It is now recognized that AF may plateau, remit/relapse, and one patient can simultaneously have multiple types of AF [5]. The ESC has also identified seven clinical types of AF, as the etiology of AF may relate to any of multiple mechanisms (see **Table 2**). In addition to types and categories of AF, the arrhythmia burden is frequently used as a metric to describe the amount of time an individual spends in AF [6].

IntechOpen

Types of AF	Definition	Treatments
First diagnosed	Newly identified AF of any type	Varies, depending on how severe the AF is and if the patient is symptomatic
Paroxysmal	Sudden onset, self-terminating episodes that typically last a few moments to as long as 48 h; recurrent	Episodes terminate with or without intervention; may be asymptomatic
Persistent	AF that lasts more than 7 days but can be converted with medical intervention	Pharmacological or electrical cardioversion
Long-standing persistent	AF that lasts a year or more and for which treatment is available	Catheter-based ablation, open ablation, drug therapy
Permanent	AF that has lasted more than a year and which is accepted by patient and medical team	Rate control

These distinctions are based primarily on the duration of AF.

Table 1.
Main types of AF as set forth by the European Society of Cardiology [3].

Clinical type	Characteristics	Comments
AF secondary to structural heart disease	May occur in patients with left-ventricular systolic or diastolic dysfunction or other forms of structural heart disease	Treatment approaches vary; anticoagulation therapy
Focal AF	AF paroxysms associated with localized triggers, such as the pulmonary veins	Pulmonary vein ablation may be considered; anticoagulation therapy
Polygenic AF	Genetic, early onset	Much remains to be elucidated about this type of AF; anticoagulation therapy
Postoperative AF	Occurs following cardiac or other surgery in patient without prior history of AF	This AF may remit on its own, may persist or progress; treatment varies
AF with atrial remodeling	AF typically associated with mitral stenosis and/or mitral valve surgery or other forms of valvular disease	Atria remodel in response to arrhythmic burden; anticoagulation therapy
Athlete's AF	AF, often paroxysmal, that occurs during intense athletic training	Appears to be related to intensity of exertion
Monogenic AF	Associated the cardiomyopathy and channelopathy	Anticoagulation therapy

Therapeutic interventions, when appropriate, are typically grouped as those involved rate control (allowing AF to continue but preventing a rapid ventricular response) or rhythm control (converting to sinus rhythm when possible).

Table 2.
Clinical types of AF as defined by the European Society of Cardiology [3].

Despite the vast healthcare resources required to manage AF, little epidemiological research has been conducted for this arrhythmia. AF can be an elusive arrhythmia and short episodes can be difficult to capture on conventional ECGs. New technological innovations, including the thumb ECG, may offer tools to help better understand this arrhythmia. The thumb ECG opens up new technological abilities to benefit patients and individual cases of AF as well as to benefit research to better understand the epidemiology and natural history of AF in real-world populations.

2. The challenge of AF epidemiology studies

The classic diagnostic assessments of AF require that documentation of the arrhythmia on a 12-lead ECG. An irregular pulse may cause a clinician to suspect AF, but the ECG is considered necessary for a diagnosis [7]. AF is characterized by irregular R-R intervals without discernible P-waves (except when the patient has concomitant atrioventricular third-degree block). About a third of all individuals with AF are asymptomatic, with silent AF or subclinical AF [8]. Even when symptoms occur, they may be infrequent or diffuse. Historically, early efforts to quantify the incidence and prevalence of AF and to better understand its potential relationship to stroke, heart failure, and other conditions were hampered by the limitations of standard ECG technology, the episodic nature of AF, and the large proportion of patients who had vague or no symptoms. Unfortunately, the first manifestation of AF may be stroke.

Recording AF on a standard 12-lead ECG assumes both that the clinician suspects that the patient has AF and that the AF will occur during the ECG recording. ECG monitoring is too elaborate and expensive for use in routine population testing, such as for epidemiological studies. Continuous ECG monitoring can be obtained in individual patients by a wearable Holter monitor, but such systems are cumbersome to patients and generate vast quantities of tracings that can be a burden to analyze. Holter monitors are typically used for 24 h or for a specific number of days, such as 7 days. Event recorders may also be used. The advent of diagnostic counters in cardiac implantable electronic devices (CIEDs) allowed physicians to monitor device-detected arrhythmias, including AF. CIED monitoring offered the advantage of beat-by-beat analysis. Clinicians could program a cutoff rate for *high rate events* on the atrial channels, usually in the lower range of 170–220 beats per minute. This led to a shift in terminology in that these devices obtained date on atrial high-rate episodes (AHRE), which included ectopic atrial tachycardia, atrial flutter, as well as AF. Current dual-chamber CIEDs offer mode-switching algorithms, which can essentially turn off ventricular tracking during episodes of AHRE. Mode-switching algorithms in conventional pacemakers can identify AHRE with 98% sensitivity and 100% specificity [9]. The value of this beat-by-beat monitoring first emerged in the Mode Selection Trial (MOST) in which 313 patients (median age 74 years) with pacemakers to treat sinus node dysfunction were followed for 27 months, during which their pacemakers recorded AHRE when atrial activity occurred at a rate > 220 beats per minute for more than 5 minutes [10]. More than half (51.3%) had AHRE, which in turn could be associated with elevated morbidity (stroke, permanent AF) and mortality [10]. The asymptomatic atrial fibrillation and stroke evaluation in pacemaker patients and atrial fibrillation reduction atrial pacing trial (ASSERT study) evaluated 2580 patients over age 65 with hypertension but without a history of AF who had a pacemaker or ICD with an atrial lead. In the first 3 months of follow-up, 10.1% of patients had documented subclinical AF lasting over 6 min; at 2.5 years, subclinical AF occurred at least once in 34.7% of patients. The patients with subclinical AF had a 2.49-fold increased risk of stroke compared to patients who did not have subclinical AF, irrespective of any other atrial arrhythmias [11]. In a study of 356 pacemaker patients with continuous atrial-channel monitoring, 88.2% had paroxysmal AF and 50.3% had at least one episode of persistent AF [12]. A study of 678 pacemaker patients (411 without AF and 267 with known AF) were followed over 38 months, and it was found that 30% of those with no history of prior AF had silent AF [13]. Of course, the patient populations for these studies were limited to those with specific device indications (and in some cases other inclusion criteria), and therefore, these findings are not generalizable to the population as a whole.

As might be intuitively expected, the accuracy of AHRE detection improves with more continuous monitoring [14]. The high prevalence of AHREs detected by device diagnostics gave rise to the implantable loop recorder (ILR). The ILR relies on a detection algorithm to identify AF typically based on R-R interval stability as evidenced by consecutive QRS complexes. AF detection algorithms in ILRs are undergoing refinement and may change in the future to improve specificity and sensitivity. As with a CIED, an ILR would be implanted only in patients who are suspected of having AF or other arrhythmias. The TRENDS study was an observational trial (n = 2486), which followed patients with an ILR for a mean of 1.4 years and analyzed them for atrial tachycardia and AF burden and thromboembolic events and found 45% of patients with no prior history of AF (n = 1988) had subclinical episodes of atrial tachycardia [15].

The incidence and prevalence of AF may be vastly underestimated because there was until recently no reliable and accurate way to monitor patients who were not at specific risk for AF or who did not have a device or ILR indication. In other words, till now, AF data were gathered mainly from people with or at an elevated risk for arrhythmias. Epidemiological information on AF progression (from paroxysmal to persistent and permanent), risk factors for AF, and AF associations remain to be elucidated. Statistical analyses and meta-analyses have allowed certain risk factors for AF to emerge, such as hypertension, heart failure, coronary artery disease, valvular disease, diabetes mellitus, obesity, and chronic renal failure [16–18] as well as risk factors for AF progression, including older age and hypertension [19]. The thumb ECG offers an excellent opportunity to gather real-world data on AF from general and specific populations. Some important questions about AF remain to be elucidated:

- What is the actual incidence and prevalence of AF in the general population?
- Are there specific subpopulations with a higher prevalence of AF, for example, patients with diabetes, myocardial infarction, and cancer patients?
- What is the association between silent AF and stroke, for example, how many patients with silent AF are needed to have one patient suffer a stroke?
- What is the trajectory of AF—does it always progress? Can we define its course in clinically meaningful ways?
- Can patients with a low AF burden plateau for a long period of time at that level or does AF typically advance to increase the AF burden?
- What can be known about the population who has more than one type of AF at the same time (for example, both paroxysmal and persistent long-standing AF)? Do multiple types of concurrent AF confer worse morbidity and mortality?
- Can we better identify risk factors for AF?

In addition to these questions, it would be important to be able to better evaluate treatment strategies for AF by monitoring patients following drug therapy, ablation, or other procedures.

3. The thumb ECG

The thumb ECG is a small-format, patient-friendly device that lay persons can use to monitor their heart rhythm. After reading the instructions or a brief training, individuals can use the thumb ECG on their own quickly and conveniently many times over the course of a day. The thumb ECG is a miniaturized and digital descendant of the original ECG technology that was available around 1900. Patients can monitor their heart rhythm by pressing the device to the chest or by placing their thumbs on pads at the top of the device for a reading (see **Figure 1**). Several thumb ECG devices are available, and it is likely more are in development. Among them, the Coala Heart Monitor™ has been approved for use in Europe to individual patients in 2016 as a Class IIa medical device and to professional organizations in 2017. The device is connected to a cloud-based service to which users subscribe. When information is uploaded from the thumb ECG to the cloud, it is automatically analyzed for AF or other arrhythmias using proprietary algorithms. Devices are available for use by multiple patients at a clinic but may also be purchased direct-to-consumer (the Coala Heart Monitor Pro™ and the Coala Heart Monitor™, respectively). The Coala device is connected via wireless Bluetooth connectivity to a smartphone for use with a proprietary Coala app. In this way, the thumb ECG dispenses with chest electrodes or other adhesive patches. An ECG may take up to 60 s.

The patient can view the individual ECG recordings and results from automated analysis directly on their smartphone app. Messages from the clinic to the patient can also be viewed directly on the app for feedback. ECG recordings can also be stored or printed by the patient to keep on hand for their next appointment. Patients can also add a special *heart report* service to their smartphone to discuss their ECG recordings with trained nurses for recommended actions. In this way, one centralized and highly specialized healthcare function may provide first-line primary cardiac healthcare coverage for a large and geographically spread-out population.

Clinicians monitor the results from their patients' thumb ECG devices by accessing a secure portal via an ordinary laptop computer. The proprietary algorithms for ECG analysis are based on the ECG Parser, an algorithm system. The ECG Parser identifies specific beats and patterns of beats and groups them into classes by

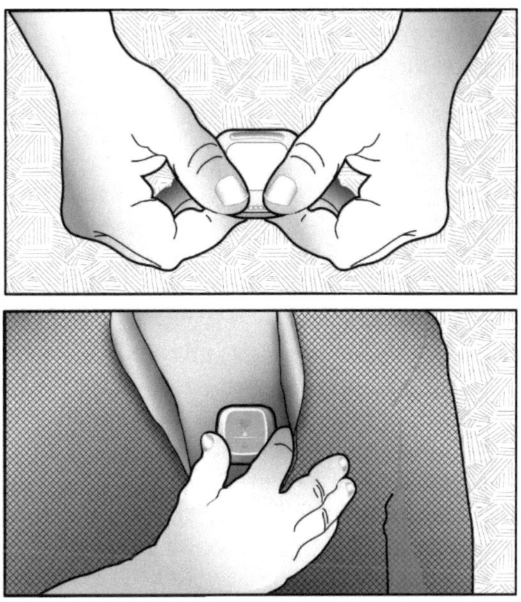

Figure 1.
The Coala Heart Monitor™. Device sensors detect the heart rhythm when the device is placed on the chest or when the device is grasped with the thumbs on top of the two sensors on the device. Drawing: Courtesy of Todd Cooper.

Category	Description	Does this indicate AF?
0	Poor quality	No
1	Normal	No
2	Atrial fibrillation	Yes
3	Pause/AV block II	No
4	Fast, regular	No
5	Long-short sequences	No
6	Bigeminy	No
7	Trigeminy	No
8	More than 5 supraventricular extrasystoles	No
9	More than 5 ventricular extrasystoles	No
10	Irregular rhythm with P-waves	No

Table 3.
The Coala Heart Monitor™ system is based on an ECG parser with a proprietary and algorithmic system to help categorize arrhythmias automatically (Category 2 events indicate AF based on R-R interval dispersion and the absence of P-waves).

morphology; using the sequence of beats, the algorithm applies markers to ranges, measures intervals based on averaged beats, and then categorizes each signal or signal segment into one of the 12 different categories to facilitate their use in large databases (see **Table 3**).

4. The role of the thumb ECG in AF research

The ability to easily and inexpensively obtain ECG data has opened up new avenues to advance research into AF and other arrhythmias.

4.1 The role of premature atrial contractions and premature ventricular contractions in arrhythmogenesis

It has long been suspected that premature atrial contractions (PACs) and premature ventricular contractions (PVCs) may be associated with arrhythmias. However, since PACs and PVCs typically occur without warning and as isolated events, there has been no way to obtain appropriate data to investigate this question without generating an overwhelming volume of tracings. A study published in 2012 attempted to explore the relationship of PACs and PVCS to AF by evaluating 428 patients without structural heart disease and with no history of AF using 24-h Holter monitoring [20]. This study found that frequent PACs were indeed significant predictors of AF ($p < 0.001$). However, the study required patients to wear Holter monitors and the investigators had to analyze hundreds of hours of ECGs. A similar study was undertaken using thumb ECG technology that could analyze 40,000 measurements over a span of 500 days. This second study was able to likewise confirm that frequent PACs were indeed highly significant predictors of AF ($p < 0.001$) [21] (see **Figure 2**).

Furthermore, with thumb ECG technology, it was relatively straightforward to confirm that the rate of VES and SVES events increased as AF developed [21] (see **Figure 3**).

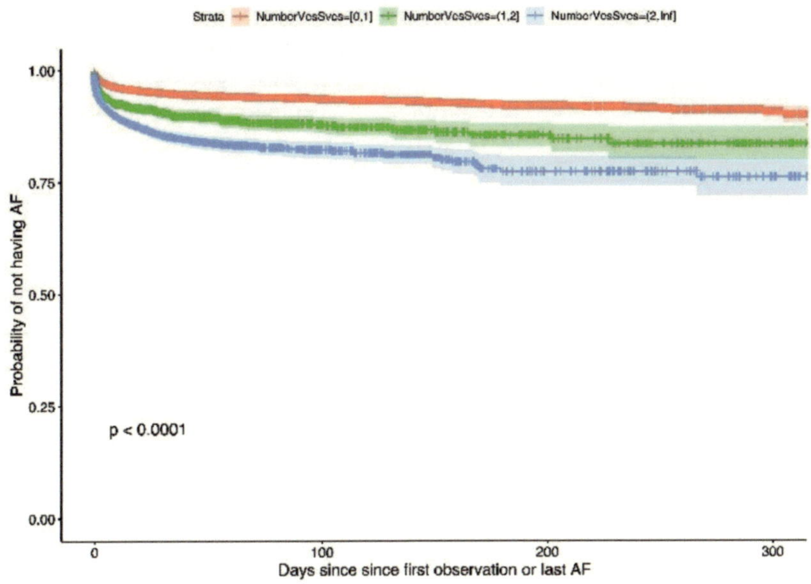

Figure 2.
The incidence rates for development of AF based on number of ventricular extrasystoles (VES) and supraventricular extrasystoles (SVES). Chart: Courtesy of Coala Life.

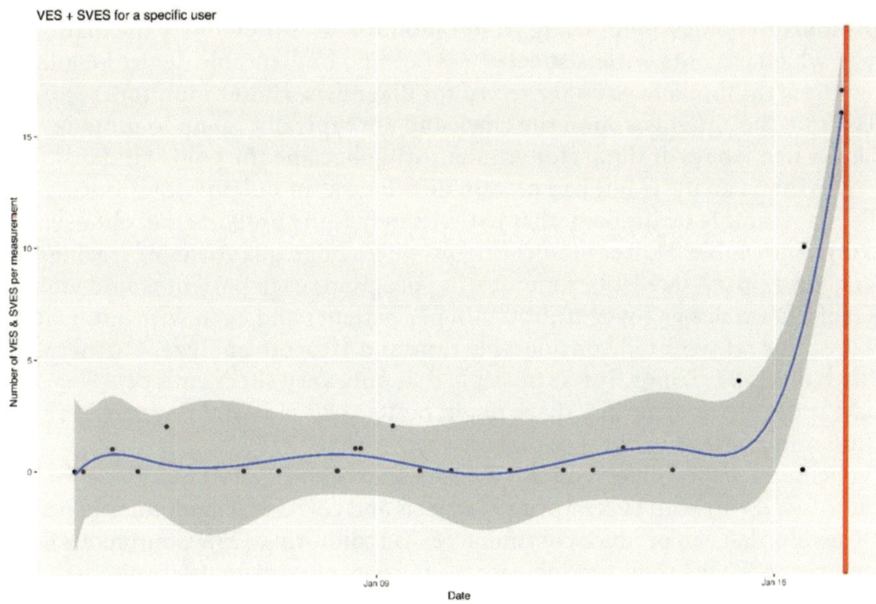

Figure 3.
As patients developed AF, the incidence of both ventricular extrasystoles and supraventricular extrasystoles increased sharply. Chart: Courtesy of Coala Life.

4.2 The real-world incidence and prevalence of AF

The StrokeStop I study was aimed at evaluating the risk of stroke in people with untreated AF. To accomplish the study, systematic ECG screenings would be needed from over 7000 patients. A thumb ECG system was used to obtain intermittent ECG recordings, which were then analyzed using a proprietary ECG parser system. In the group of patients aged 75 or 76 years, AF prevalence was found to be 12.3% [22]. This differs markedly from medical records, which found that in that particular patient group, 9.3% had a prior diagnosis of AF. Thus, thumb ECG with the ECG parser technology was able to confirm a much higher AF prevalence than was previously determined. This suggests that the actual incidence and prevalence of real-world AF may be substantially underestimated, which has implications for public health and the healthcare system as well as for individual patients.

In the ongoing *Study of Men Born in 1943*, thumb ECGs were introduced in 2014 to help assess AF prevalence. After eliminating patients who had died, declined to participate, were lost to follow-up, or had known permanent AF, patients were evaluated twice daily by thumb ECG (n = 479). The thumb ECG in this study was able to diagnose a previously silent form of AF in 1.8% of patients (n = 8), and it found the overall prevalence of AF was 3.1% (95% confidence interval [CI], 1.83 to 4.98), but for men over the age of 71, the prevalence of paroxysmal AF was 9.9% [23].

In a study of 1510 patients aged 65 with risk factors for stroke, the use of thumb ECGs over a two-week period found undiagnosed AF in 0.9% of the population, which worked out for a total AF prevalence in the study group of 7.6% [24].

5. Thumb ECGs versus other types of monitoring

Ambulatory assessment using Holter monitors was previously the main way in which patients with suspected AF (and no implantable device) could allow the arrhythmia to *go on the record* for diagnosis. Holter monitors record ECGs from the patient around the clock and are typically set up to provide either 24 h or 7 days of data. Holter monitoring became the gold standard for arrhythmia analysis but had certain drawbacks: ambulatory monitoring utilizes a wearable technology that patients may find cumbersome, clumsy, and uncomfortable. Holter monitoring produces huge quantities of tracings to be analyzed. In a 7-day Holter monitoring program, each patient would yield 168 h of ECG tracings (over 10,000 min per patient) and even with automated systems, this represented considerable time and effort to analyze. Furthermore, in 168 h of ECG tracings, it was possible that only very short runs of AF would appear—for example, there might be 10 or 20 min of AF somewhere in 10,000 min of data.

Subclinical device-detected AF is defined as an AHRE (>190 beats/min for >6 min and <24 h) with lack of prior diagnosis and correlated symptoms in patients with devices that can produce continuous ECG monitoring [25]. Continuous ECG monitoring has been shown to increase the number of undiagnosed episodes of AF, especially in those with prior bouts of ischemia [26]. In fact, thumb (or handheld) ECGs have been shown to be significantly more sensitive in the detection of silent AF compared to conventional 24-h Holter ECGs [27, 28].

In order to determine whether Holter monitors offered comparable efficacy to thumb ECGs, a study of 95 patients (≥65 years) was initiated. Patients were excluded if they had a history of AF. All patients were monitored for 5 days using a Holter monitor and concurrently with a thumb ECG twice daily. Patients continued using the thumb ECG for 30 days. Paroxysmal AF was detected in 20 patients using the thumb ECG, in 17 patients using the Holter monitor, and by both systems in 10 patients [29]. The detection rates between the two methods did not differ in a statistically significant way (p = 0.63).

DOI: http://dx.doi.org/10.5772/intechopen.83660

In a study of 108 consecutive patients with ambiguous symptoms of dizziness and heart palpitations, patients were monitored using a Holter monitor for 24 h and then twice daily using a thumb ECG for 28 days. The mean age of patients in this study was 54.1 years. In this study, the thumb ECG was significantly more effective over 4 weeks at identifying AF and paroxysmal supraventricular tachycardia than the Holter monitor [30].

In a study presented at the Cardiovascular Spring Meeting in Stockholm in April 2018, researchers took 1000 consecutive, anonymous printouts of waveforms captured from the chest and thumbs using the Coala Heart Monitor™ system. No exclusions were allowed. Each printout consisted of three 10-s tracings recorded at 25 mm/s. Algorithm analysis notation and patient information (except patient sex and age by 10-year groups) were removed from the strips. However, heart rate, R-R median values, and user-provided annotations were allowed. All strips came from real-world patients using the Coala monitor; subjects were given no special device training. All strips were then sent to a trained cardiologist who interpreted each one manually and then compared his interpretation to the automatic analysis offered by the Coala device. One cardiologist interpreted all of the rhythm strips. When comparing these 1000 real-world ECGs to the Coala algorithm's interpretation, it was found that the Coala was highly accurate with 97% sensitivity and 95% specificity. The estimated prevalence of AF from these recordings was 14.4% [31, 32].

In the StrokeStop I study, 80,149 tracings were recorded using the Zenicor™ thumb ECG system; tracings were obtained from 3209 patients aged 75 or 76 years. It was found to offer 98% sensitivity and 88% specificity, and the use of thumb ECG technology combined with an ECG parser reduced the workload in analyzing data by over 85% [22].

In a study of 100 patients with AF, a 12-lead ECG recording was followed by a thumb ECG assessment with the results compared by a blinded investigator. When the 12-lead ECG was compared to the thumb ECG, the thumb ECG had a sensitivity of 96% and a specificity of 92% versus the 12-lead ECG. As part of the same study, a second group of patients (n = 12) underwent effective cardioversion for AF and then used a thumb ECG to assess their rhythms twice a day for the next 30 days. In this group, 95% of cardioverted patients had tracings from the thumb ECG considered to be of sufficient quality for clinical diagnosis. A third group (n = 606) was screened for AF using the thumb ECG. Twelve people in this group were diagnosed with AF of whom six had no history of AF and no symptoms [33].

6. Questions about silent AF

One of the primary reasons to suspect that AF incidence and prevalence is underestimated is the fact that as much as 40% of AF may be asymptomatic [34, 35]. Clinically silent AF may occur with paroxysmal AF, persistent long-standing AF, or permanent AF [36]. Asymptomatic AF is not benign; data from the EORP-AF study found that asymptomatic AF conferred on patients a higher 1-year mortality risk than symptomatic AF [35] although the AFFIRM study found no such difference between symptomatic and asymptomatic AF patients [37]. Early and accurate diagnosis of AF may help reduce the burden of AF on the healthcare system and may allow interventions to reduce morbidity and mortality associated with AF.

The classic AF symptoms may include any or a combination of the following: heart palpitations, sensations of a racing or pounding heart, dyspnea, chest pain or discomfort, fatigue, lethargy, dizziness, malaise, anxiety, and syncope. Symptoms are thought to be caused primarily by rapid ventricular response to AF rather than by the atrial arrhythmia itself. It is thought that rapid ventricular activity, irregular rhythms, and the loss of the atrial contribution to ventricular filling might all contribute to reduced cardiac output, exacerbation of left-ventricular dysfunction, cardiac remodeling, and a general deterioration of overall health [36]. In addition to asymptomatic paroxysmal AF, some cases of AF may go unnoticed by patients because the AF episodes are brief and interspersed between long periods of normal sinus rhythm and symptoms may be very mild, diffuse, or overlooked by patients. Silent AF is typically an incidental diagnosis, which may occur during routine examinations or tests for other conditions.

The mechanical effects on the heart caused by fibrillating atria as well as the electrophysiological and neurological consequences of AF appear to be the same whether AF is clinically silent or symptomatic. Silent AF, like its symptomatic counterpart, is associated with silent or symptomatic emboli, heart failure, morbidity, and mortality [38].

Risk factors for silent AF include patients with cryptogenic stroke, hypertension, advanced age, obesity, diabetes mellitus, cigarette smoking, chronic kidney disease, or a history of cardiac disease [7, 35, 39–42]. Blood group type 0 appears to confer a protective effect against thromboembolism in persons with AF for reasons that remain unclear, but which may be associated with circulating von Willebrand factor levels [43].

7. Anticoagulation therapy

AF has been clearly associated with the catastrophic complications of thromboembolism and cerebral stroke, but the association between AHRE and thromboembolism/stroke is not well defined [44]. The thumb ECG, like CIEDs, can detect AHRE but it remains an open question as to whether and under what circumstances anticoagulation therapy is appropriate for patients with documented AHRE. AHRE is defined by two parameters: the atrial rate and the duration of the episode. However, it remains unclear as to how fast or how long an episode of AHRE must be to represent a risk of thromboembolism or stroke [45]. Thus, it remains to be elucidated at which point a patient with AHRE might benefit from anticoagulation therapy.

According to the ASSERT and TRENDS studies, the association between the formation of a thromboembolism and AHRE is challenged by the lack of a temporal relation between the two events [46, 47]. The current data are contradictory. In the ASSERT study, tachyarrhythmic episodes ≥6 min in duration have led to a higher embolic risk [11]. However, in the TRENDS study, tachyarrhythmic episodes ≤5.5 h were not associated with an increased thromboembolic risk [15].

With much to be elucidated about the potential role of anticoagulation therapy for patients with AHRE, thumb ECGs may play an important role. These devices may help uncover more about AHRE and its relationship to AF as well as its association to adverse events. A more refined understanding of the temporal relationship between AF and its comorbidities will help to create more effective anticoagulation therapies and better outcomes.

8. Knowledge gaps about AF

The incidence and prevalence of AF may correlate with gender, age, comorbidities (such as heart failure, atherosclerosis, hypertension, diabetes mellitus, and others), and possibly other variables. The natural course of AF, once thought to be the linear progression from paroxysmal to persistent to permanent, remains to be elucidated and appears to be more fluid than originally thought, even allowing for remission and relapsing. While the association between AF and stroke is clear and ominous, it is not known if this risk is greater, lesser, or the same for symptomatic versus asymptomatic AF or different types or clinical presentations of AF. A meta-analysis of data on AF showed that while men generally had a higher incidence of AF than women, women and, in particular elderly women, were at a greater risk than men for stroke and thromboembolism associated with AF [48–50]. Whether or not AF in the elderly and oldest old populations is associated with more or more severe symptoms also remains unknown. Greater understanding of these matters could result in better, more targeted, and more effective clinical approaches and treatment.

It has been observed that patients implanted with CIEDs may experience brief, clinically silent episodes of paroxysmal AF when the device is initially implanted. The Automatic Interpretation for Diagnosis Assistance (AIDA) study found that half (50.6%) of patients with *de novo* pacemaker implantations experienced atrial arrhythmias in the first month following implant and these episodes were often asymptomatic [51]. In a study of 213 dual-chamber pacemaker patients, all of them had experienced at least one atrial arrhythmia at 3 years following implant [52]. This area has not been studied extensively and it is not known if this is clinically important or might resolve with time [53].

Other knowledge gaps occur in the treatment of AF and how patients respond. It has been suggested that pharmacological suppression of AF may simply convert symptomatic AF into clinically silent AF, but there is not much data to support or refute this notion. While it is known that AF incidence and prevalence increases with age, it is not clear whether geriatric patients are more likely to have symptomatic or asymptomatic AF, nor has it been fully elucidated whether certain types of AF (such as permanent or persistent long-standing AF) occur more often in elderly patients.

AF is thought to be more prevalent in industrialized nations compared to developing countries but this has not been extensively studied [54].

Thumb ECG studies can provide robust data to help answer these questions by allowing the inexpensive and straightforward acquisition of large amounts of ECG data annotated with patient-reported symptoms from selected populations and, together with algorithms to analyze the data, provide for fast and accurate interpretation of that data. The advent of thumb ECG technology will empower medical science and the healthcare system to obtain vital information crucial to the early and accurate diagnosis of AF, particularly paroxysmal and clinically silent AF.

Thumb ECG data may help better guide anticoagulation therapy. Anticoagulation therapy is frequently prescribed for AF patients. In CIED patients with diagnostic data revealing atrial high-rate activity, it is not clear despite this documentation whether patients would benefit from anticoagulation therapy [38].

The populations affected by AF are diverse and include patients with valvular disease, malignancy, inflammation, atherosclerotic coronary artery disease, plus those with genetic forms of AF, postoperative patients, patients following ablations, CIED patients, along with patients who are geriatric, obese, or who have heart failure and/or hypertension. These populations are diverse, some overlap considerably, and cross the lines between medical disciplines [40]. These factors contribute to the confusion that makes it hard to better quantify AF. A number of open questions remain and a high-level summary appears in **Table 4**.

Question	Obstacles	Comments
Which patient populations are at greatest risk from AF?	May require some kind of diagnostic algorithm to account for comorbidities; need to find definition of risk (risk of AF, stroke, mortality).	Likewise, an important unanswered question is which populations are at lowest risk? Why?
Can patients use thumb ECG technology to self-monitor and/or collect data?	Requires study parameters to be set up.	May be most helpful means to get more accurate and comprehensive AF data.
What is the normal trajectory of AF?	Requires more data, also it is not clear if the natural course of AF might vary by population (for instance, it might be different in older than younger patients, or in men versus women).	The old paradigm that *AF begets AF* may not be true or may be only partially accurate.
Are some types of AF associated with greater morbidity and mortality than others?	Requires more data and possibly stratification.	This question could lead to more individualized treatment courses.
Can we reach a consensus definition for AF burden?	This is a relatively new term that is typically well understood but imperfectly quantified; need consensus definition.	It is not clear if and in what ways AF burden may relate to AF risks/outcomes. Once it is defined, it can be more efficiently studied.
Is silent AF always without symptoms?	Evidence that quality of life decreases in patients even with asymptomatic AF suggests that AF is almost always symptomatic but not all symptoms are recognized.	Better diagnostic tools are needed to identify silent AF and then to measure quality of life.
What is actual incidence and prevalence of AF?	Correlations with clinical presentation, type, history, duration, and patient characteristics may be helpful but challenging to obtain.	Will allow for more effective and individually targeted treatments.

Table 4.
Key questions about AF that may be a good research topic with thumb ECG technology [40].

9. The AF burden and thumb ECG technology

In an effort to better grapple with the global effects of AF on a patient, the AF burden is often used to better describe the arrhythmia and its consequences. The AF burden may be defined as how much time the patient spends in AF per unit of time (such as what proportion of 1 day or 1 week) [6]. AF burden lacks a universally recognized consensus definition, has not been extensively validated as a measure, and is not often used when evaluating AF cases in terms of severity or risk. It is not known if a high AF burden exacerbates risk factors for stroke. It is strongly suspected that the AF burden is generally underestimated because of asymptomatic AF and the fact that conventional technologies have been used to assess the incidence and prevalence of AF [38]. A consensus definition would be helpful and would facilitate meaningful efforts to study how the AF burden affects the course of the arrhythmia, treatment options, and related morbidity and mortality.

10. An integrated approach to care for AF patients using thumb ECG technology

A knowledge deficit about AF may be observed even in patients provided specific, patient-focused oral, and/or written educational tools [55, 56]. Individualized, educational interventions for AF have been proposed in order to address specific patient needs, for example, types of AF treatment, recommended lifestyle modifications, possible self-management tools, and drug therapy [57]. Thumb ECG technology may soon emerge as an important element in the care of AF patients. Patients who are considered appropriate candidates to monitor their hearts using a thumb ECG device should be given specific training on the use of the device; such training would likely be brief as these devices are designed to be easy to use for laypeople. The regular use of a thumb ECG can assist patients in arrhythmia detection and diagnosis as well as monitoring the course of treatment. The integration of the thumb ECG into AF patient care may empower the patient and be a cornerstone of a shared decision-making paradigm, in the event that multiple treatment options are considered. It is known that patient education, shared accountability, and individual empowerment drive improved adherence [58]. The use of a thumb ECG may also be helpful in linking AF episodes to specific symptoms [3]. Furthermore, the thumb ECG may reveal subclinical AF and may help better delineate the progression of AF over time.

AF is so pervasive and crosses so many disciplinary boundaries that a multidisciplinary approach to care is warranted, bringing together several healthcare disciplines, i.e., general practitioners, cardiologists, surgeons, and allied health professionals along with nonspecialists who may advise on diet, lifestyle modifications, physical and occupational therapy, and stroke prevention tactics. Moreover, patients with newly diagnosed AF may benefit from a comprehensive cardiovascular evaluation, including transthoracic echocardiography, as they are at risk for other cardiovascular conditions [59, 60].

AF treatment typically involves anticoagulation therapy (initiated early in appropriate patients), lifestyle modifications, and appropriate interventions, which could include the use of antiarrhythmic agents or other pharmacological treatments, catheter-based interventions, or surgical procedures (ablation, left atrial appendage occluders, etc.) [3]. Growing understanding of how altered calcium homeostasis, atrial fibrosis, ion-channel dysfunction, autonomic imbalance, and oxidative stress may contribute to AF combined with new knowledge about the genetic underpinnings of arrhythmias should all be taken into account when structuring AF care programs [61]. As an example, pulmonary vein ablation has been recommended for some types of AF but would not benefit all AF patients. However, all AF patients are likely to benefit from regular, consistent, systematic care including routine follow-up visits, monitoring overall physical condition, arrhythmia assessments, pharmacological adjustments as needed, and assessments and encouragement to promote treatment adherence. Thumb ECG monitoring would be an integral part of that care paradigm.

AF care can be defined by three broad domains: stroke prevention (anticoagulation therapy), rate control (mainly aimed at symptomatic improvement), and rhythm control (arrhythmia conversion). Pharmacological therapy can be an important element of AF care and varies based on the individual characteristics of the patient (age, target for treatment, comorbidities, symptoms, symptom severity, left-ventricular ejection fraction, hemodynamics, other drugs the patient may be taking, and so on). Acute rhythm control can be achieved pharmacologically in up to half of all patients diagnosed with recent-onset AF by using antiarrhythmic agents. Antiarrhythmic drug therapy should be guided first by safety rather than effectiveness, and treatment goals should be established that seek symptomatic improvement with the foreknowledge that side effects with these drugs are common [3]. Dose reduction of antiarrhythmic agents may be needed for geriatric patients in that metabolism and the heart's electrical system slow down with increasing age [62]. Above all, it should be noted that many antiarrhythmic agents have seemingly paradoxical pro-arrhythmic effects. This requires regular ECG monitoring to protect patients against the onset of a new drug-induced arrhythmia [63]. While there are to date no studies on the role of thumb ECG technology in this setting, it makes intuitive sense that a thumb ECG may be useful for patients on antiarrhythmic drug therapy.

11. Future directions

The usefulness of the Coala Heart Monitor™ needs further validation with regard to specific patient groups. Currently, the TEASE study is evaluating patients with cryptogenic stroke for 28 days using the Coala Heart Monitor™ [64]. The rationale for prolonged monitoring in this population is warranted in order to determine if anticoagulation is indicated. Furthermore, the Red Heart Study is an initiative using the Coala Heart Monitor™ exclusively among women with suspected AF or other arrhythmias [65].

While the thumb ECG has already proven its value as a tool for finding and following the progression of AF and other arrhythmias, it is beyond the functionality of this device to assess structural heart changes or impaired left-ventricular function. However, some thumb ECG devices already on the market, such as the Coala Heart Monitor™, have the capacity to record simultaneously both chest ECG and heart sounds through an electronic stethoscope membrane. This allows derivation of acoustic cardiographic parameters such as systolic time intervals (STI) along with the presence and intensity of S3 and S4 heart sounds. The use of STI has historically proven to be a highly sensitive method of assessment of changes in left-ventricular function, albeit with inconclusive findings as a diagnostic tool for differential diagnosis [66, 67].

The use of acoustic cardiographic parameters derived from repeated patient-engaged recordings performed in the home environment may, in this way, characterize and track changes in left-ventricular function at low cost and low burden to the healthcare system. Such indicative parameters of change in cardiac function may fully utilize the individualized data collected from many recordings over a period of time as a baseline rather than population-derived and regression-corrected baseline data for improved sensitivity and accuracy.

In the future, the automatic algorithm-driven detection and reporting of sudden deviations in the patient's heart rhythm may help reduce the human workload without compromising care, in that the healthcare provider at the clinic can be notified quickly about these deviations and take appropriate action, such as changing medications. It is plausible that this could all happen before the patient experiences any symptoms. In this way, small, highly specialized healthcare centers may provide first-line cardiac primary healthcare coverage with respect to AF or AF with left-ventricular dysfunction (e.g., decompensated heart failure) for a large and geographically widespread patient population. These centers would be centralized in terms of their function, but not necessarily geographically centralized.

Centralized data processing, ultimately with data from possibly millions of recordings, may provide for high detection accuracy and is an ideal application for machine learning or artificial intelligence, which could utilize pattern-recognition algorithms on these datasets to provide an early indication of any characteristic pathological developments, which can then be confirmed or ruled out in a traditional healthcare setting using conventional techniques and modalities. Continuous patient feedback through the smartphone, potentially even using *gamification* to create a game-type application, may improve patient engagement and adherence to proposed lifestyle or dietary changes and pharmacological compliance. This platform may also be an ideal tool for running very large cost-effective clinical studies, in that data collection can take place using the thumb ECG. Patients can use the device and the smartphone app in the privacy of their own homes to track their own results and monitor symptoms. This could likely be done at a very low cost with few technical or logistical barriers. While visionary in concept, such a system may provide a unique solution for improved patient outcomes through early intervention and close follow-up of treatment with potential (and substantial) reductions in cost and resource utilization to the healthcare system.

12. Conclusions

AF is a prevalent arrhythmia that poses a significant burden on the healthcare system, but it is under-diagnosed in that it can be challenging to capture the arrhythmia on a 12-lead ECG (required for diagnosis), and up to a third of patients are asymptomatic. The thumb ECG offers an innovative, user-friendly approach to consistent cardiac self-monitoring that may provide new insights into the incidence and prevalence of AF. The use of pattern-recognition algorithms, artificial intelligence, and smartphone apps may allow the thumb ECG both to facilitate care for cardiac patients in the future and to make large studies of arrhythmias more cost effective.

Conflict of interest

MS is employed by Coala Life AB, Stockholm, Sweden. The other authors have no conflict of interests.

Thanks

We acknowledge Todd Cooper for **Figure 1** and Mattias Jönsson for providing the charts.

Author details

Peter Magnusson[1,2], Magnus Samuelsson[3], Joseph V. Pergolizzi Jr [4,5], Hani Annabi[5] and Jo Ann LeQuang[5]*

1 Cardiology Research Unit, Department of Medicine, Karolinska Institute, Stockholm, Sweden

2 Centre for Research and Development, Uppsala University/Region Gävleborg, Sweden

3 Coala Life AB, Stockholm, Sweden

4 Native Cardio Inc., Naples, Florida, USA

5 NEMA Research Inc., Naples, Florida, USA

*Address all correspondence to: joann@leqmedical.com

References

[1] Association AHAaAS. When the Beat is Off–Atrial Fibrillation. American Heart Association and American Stroke Association. 2016. Available from: /www.strokeassociation.org/STROKEORG/LifeAfterStroke/HealthyLivingAfterStroke/UnderstandingRiskyConditions/When-the-Beat-is-Off---Atrial-Fibrillation_UCM_310782_Article.jsp#.W8o1TWhKiUk [Accessed: November 27, 2019]

[2] Kotecha D, Piccini J. Atrial fibrillation in heart failure: What should we do? European Heart Journal. 2015;**36**(46):3250-3257. DOI: 10.1093eurheartj/ehv513

[3] Kirchhof P, Benussi S, Kotecha D, Ahlsson A, Atar D, Casadei B, et al. 2016 ESC Guidelines for the management of atrial fibrillation developed in collaboration with EACTS. European Heart Journal. 2016;**37**(38):2893-2962. DOI: 10.1093/eurheartj/ehw210

[4] Jahangir A, Lee V, Friedman PA, Trusty JM, Hodge DO, Kopecky SL, et al. Long-term progression and outcomes with aging in patients with lone atrial fibrillation: A 30-year follow-up study. Circulation. 2007;**115**(24):3050-3056

[5] Sugihara C, Veasey R, Freemantle N, Podd S, Furniss S, Sulke N. The development of AF over time in patients with permanent pacemakers: Objective assessment with pacemaker diagnostics demonstrates distinct patterns of AF. Europace. 2015;**17**(6):864-870. DOI: 10.1093/europace/euv032

[6] Passman R, Bernstein RA. New appraisal of atrial fibrillation burden and stroke prevention. Stroke. 2016;**47**(2):570-576. DOI: 10.1161/STROKEAHA.115.009930

[7] January CT, Wann LS, Alpert JS, Calkins H, Cigarroa JE, Cleveland JC Jr, et al. 2014 AHA/ACC/HRS guideline for the management of patients with atrial fibrillation: Executive summary: A report of the American College of Cardiology/American Heart Association Task Force on practice guidelines and the Heart Rhythm Society. Circulation. 2014;**130**(23):2071-2104

[8] Healey JS, Alings M, Ha A, Leong-Sit P, Birnie DH, de Graaf JJ, et al. Subclinical atrial fibrillation in older patients. Circulation. 2017;**136**(14):1276-1283

[9] Passman RS, Weinberg KM, Freher M, Denes P, Schaechter A, Goldberger JJ, et al. Accuracy of mode switch algorithms for detection of atrial tachyarrhythmias. Journal of Cardiovascular Electrophysiology. 2004;**15**(7):773-777

[10] Glotzer T, Hellkamp A, Zimmerman J, Sweeney M, Yee R, Marinchak R, et al. Atrial high rate episodes detected by pacemaker diagnostics predict death and stroke. Circulation. 2003;**107**:1614-1619

[11] Healey JS, Connolly SJ, Gold MR, Israel CW, Van Gelder IC, Capucci A, et al. Subclinical atrial fibrillation and the risk of stroke. The New England Journal of Medicine. 2012;**366**(2):120-129. DOI: 10.1056/NEJMoa1105575

[12] Veasey RA, Sugihara C, Sandhu K, Dhillon G, Freemantle N, Furniss SS, et al. The natural history of atrial fibrillation in patients with permanent pacemakers: Is atrial fibrillation a progressive disease? Journal of Interventional Cardiac Electrophysiology. 2015;**44**(1):23-30. DOI: 10.1007/s10840-015-0029-x

[13] Sandgren E, Rorsman C, Edvardsson N, Engdahl J. Stroke incidence and anticoagulation treatment in patients with pacemaker-detected

silent atrial fibrillation. PLoS One. 2018;**13**(9):e0203661. DOI: 10.1371/journal.pone.0203661

[14] Ziegler PD, Koehler JL, Mehra R. Comparison of continuous versus intermittent monitoring of atrial arrhythmias. Heart Rhythm. 2006;**3**(12):1445-1452

[15] Glotzer TV, Daoud EG, Wyse DG, Singer DE, Ezekowitz MD, Hilker C, et al. The relationship between daily atrial tachyarrhythmia burden from implantable device diagnostics and stroke risk: The TRENDS study. Circulation. Arrhythmia and Electrophysiology. 2009;**2**(5):474-480. DOI: 10.1161/CIRCEP.109.849638

[16] Oldgren J, Healey JS, Ezekowitz M, Commerford P, Avezum A, Pais P, et al. Variations in cause and management of atrial fibrillation in a prospective registry of 15,400 emergency department patients in 46 countries: The RE-LY Atrial Fibrillation Registry. Circulation. 2014;**129**(15):1568-1576. DOI: 10.1161/CIRCULATIONAHA.113.005451

[17] Nguyen TN, Hilmer SN, Cumming RG. Review of epidemiology and management of atrial fibrillation in developing countries. International Journal of Cardiology. 2013;**167**(6):2412-2420. DOI: 10.1016/ijcard.2013.01.184

[18] Kannel WB, Wolf PA, Benjamin EJ, Levy D. Prevalence, incidence, prognosis, and predisposing conditions for atrial fibrillation: Population-based estimates. The American Journal of Cardiology. 1998;**82**(8a):2n-9n

[19] Blum S, Meyre P, Aeschbacher S, Berger S, Auberson C, Briel M, et al. Incidence and predictors of atrial fibrillation progression: A systematic review and meta-analysis. Heart Rhythm. 24 October 2018. pii: S1547-5271(18)31049-X. DOI: 10.1016/j.hrthm.2018.10.022. [Epub ahead of print]

[20] Chong BH, Pong V, Lam KF, Liu S, Zuo ML, Lau YF, et al. Frequent premature atrial complexes predict new occurrence of atrial fibrillation and adverse cardiovascular events. Europace. 2012;**14**(7):942-947. DOI: 10.1093/europace/eur389

[21] Coala Life. Study [Clinical study]. Unpublished. 2018

[22] Svennberg E, Engdahl J, Al-Khalili F, Friberg L, Frykman V, Rosenqvist M. Mass screening for untreated atrial fibrillation: The STROKESTOP study. Circulation. 2015;**131**(25):2176-2184. DOI: 10.1161/CIRCULATIONAHA.116.026693

[23] Mandalenakis Z, Lennartsson ST, Fu M, Lappas G, Li S, Rosengren A, et al. The incidence of atrial fibrillation and the added value of thumb ECG for detecting new cases. Scandinavian Cardiovascular Journal. 2018;**10**:1-6. DOI: 10.1080/14017431/2018.1509120

[24] Berge T, Brynildsen J, Larssen HKN, Onarheim S, Jenssen GR, Ihle-Hansen H, et al. Systematic screening for atrial fibrillation in a 65-year-old population with risk factors for stroke: Data from the Akershus Cardiac Examination 1950 study. Europace. 2017;**19**(S3):iii355. DOI: 10.1093/ehjci/eux159.003

[25] Gorenek BC, Bax J, Boriani G, Chen SA, Dagres N, Glotzer TV, et al. Device-detected subclinical atrial tachyarrhythmias: Definition, implications and management—An European Heart Rhythm Association (EHRA) consensus document, endorsed by Heart Rhythm Society (HRS), Asia Pacific Heart Rhythm Society (APHRS) and Sociedad Latinoamericana de Estimulacion Cardiaca y Electrofisiologia (SOLEACE). Europace. 2017;**19**(9):1556-1578. DOI: 10.1093/europase/eux163

[26] Roche F, Gaspoz JM, Da Costa A, Isaaz K, Duverney D, Pichot V, et al. Frequent and prolonged asymptomatic episodes of paroxysmal atrial fibrillation revealed by automatic long-term event recorders in patients with a negative 24-hour Holter. Pacing and Clinical Electrophysiology. 2002;**25**(11):1587-1593

[27] Doliwa PS, Rosenqvist M, Frykman V. Paroxysmal atrial fibrillation with silent episodes: Intermittent versus continuous monitoring. Scandinavian Cardiovascular Journal. 2012;**46**(3):144-148. DOI: 10.3109/14017431.2012.661873

[28] Doliwa Sobocinski P, Anggardh Rooth E, Frykman Kull V, von Arbin M, Wallen H, Rosenqvist M. Improved screening for silent atrial fibrillation after ischaemic stroke. Europace. 2012;**14**(8):1112-1116. DOI: 10.1093/europace/eur431

[29] Poulsen MB, Binici Z, Dominguez H, Soja AM, Kruuse C, Hornnes AH, et al. Performance of short ECG recordings twice daily to detect paroxysmal atrial fibrillation in stroke and transient ischemic attack patients. International Journal of Stroke. 2017;**12**(2):192-196. DOI: 10.1177/1747493016669883

[30] Hendrikx T, Rosenqvist M, Wester P, Sandstrom H, Hornsten R. Intermittent short ECG recording is more effective than 24-hour Holter ECG in detection of arrhythmias. BMC Cardiovascular Disorders. 2014;**14**:41. DOI: 10.1186/1471-2261-14-41

[31] Olsson A. Performance evaluation of automatic symptom-ruled, real-world arrhythmic recordings. Stockholm: Sweden; 2018. Contract No.: Poster 68

[32] Olsson A. Abstract 12893: Symptom-ruled real world arrhythmic recordings with an internet based system. Circulation. 2018;**138**:A127893

[33] Doliwa PS, Frykman V, Rosenqvist M. Short-term ECG for out of hospital detection of silent atrial fibrillation episodes. Scandinavian Cardiovascular Journal. 2009;**43**(3):163-168. DOI: 10.1080/14017430802593435

[34] Ganapathy AV, Monjazeb S, Ganapathy KS, Shanoon F, Razavi M. "Asymptomatic" persistent or permanent atrial fibrillation: A misnomer in selected patients. International Journal of Cardiology. 2015;**185**:112-113. DOI: 10.1016/j.ijcard.2015.03.122

[35] Boriani G, Laroche CM, Diemberger I, Fatecchi E, Popescu M, Rasmussen L, et al. Asymptomatic atrial fibrillation: Clinical correlates, management, and outcomes in the EORP-AF Pilot General Registry. The American Journal of Medicine. 2015;**128**:509-518. DOI: 10.1016/j.amjmed.2014.11.026

[36] Savelieva I, Camm AJ. Silent atrial fibrillation—Another Pandora's box. Pacing and Clinical Electrophysiology. 2000;**23**(2):145-148

[37] Flaker GC, Belew K, Beckman K, Vidaillet H, Kron J, Safford R, et al. Asymptomatic atrial fibrillation: Demographic features and prognostic information from the Atrial Fibrillation Follow-Up Investigation of Rhythm Management (AFFIRM) study. American Heart Journal. 2005;**149**(4):657-663

[38] Dilaveris PE, Kennedy HL. Silent atrial fibrillation: Epidemiology, diagnosis, and clinical impact. Clinical Cardiology. 2017;**40**(6):413-418. DOI: 10.1002/clc/22667

[39] Camm AJ, Kirchhof P, Lip GY, Schotten U, Savelieva I, Ernst S, et al. Guidelines for the management of atrial fibrillation: The task force for the management of atrial fibrillation of the European Society of Cardiology (ESC). European Heart Journal.

2010;**31**(19):2369-2429. DOI: 10.1093/eurheartj/ehq278

[40] Kennedy HL. Silent atrial fibrillation: Definition, clarification, and unanswered issues. Annals of Noninvasive Electrocardiology. 2015;**20**(6):518-525. DOI: 10.1111/anec.12307

[41] Marfella R, Sasso FC, Siniscalchi M, Cirillo M, Paolisso P, Sardu C, et al. Brief episodes of silent atrial fibrillation predict clinical vascular brain disease in type 2 diabetic patients. Journal of the American College of Cardiology. 2013;**62**(6):525-530. DOI: 10.1016/j.jacc/2013.02.091

[42] Boriani G, Padeletti L. Management of atrial fibrillation in bradyarrhythmias. Nature Reviews. Cardiology. 2015;**12**(6):337-349. DOI: 10.1038/nrcardio.2015.30

[43] Blustin JM, McBane RD, Mazur M, Ammash N, Sochor O, Grill DE, et al. The association between thromboembolic complications and blood group in patients with atrial fibrillation. Mayo Clinic Proceedings. 2015;**90**(2):216-223. DOI: 10.1016/j.mayocp.2014.11.013

[44] Benezet-Mazuecos J, Rubio JM, Cortes M, Iglesias JA, Calle S, de la Vieja JJ, et al. Silent ischaemic brain lesions related to atrial high rate episodes in patients with cardiac implantable electronic devices. Europace. 2015;**17**(3):364-369. DOI: 10.1093/europace/euu267

[45] Surapaneni P, Safadi A, Contractor T, Patel MB, Thakur RK. Device-detected atrial fibrillation-perils and pitfalls: An update. Cardiology Clinics. 2016;**34**(2):299-306. DOI: 10.1016/j.ccl.2015.12.007

[46] Daoud EG, Glotzer TV, Wyse DG, Ezekowitz MD, Hilker C, Koehler J, et al. Temporal relationship of atrial tachyarrhythmias, cerebrovascular events, and systemic emboli based on stored device data: A subgroup analysis of TRENDS. Heart Rhythm. 2011;**8**(9):1416-1423. DOI: 10.1016/j.hrthm.2011.04.022

[47] Martin DT, Bersohn MM, Waldo AL, Wathen MS, Choucair WK, Lip GY, et al. Randomized trial of atrial arrhythmia monitoring to guide anticoagulation in patients with implanted defibrillator and cardiac resynchronization devices. European Heart Journal. 2015;**36**(26):1660-1668. DOI: 10.1093/eurheartj/ehv115

[48] Xiong Q, Proietti M, Senoo K, Lip GY. Asymptomatic versus symptomatic atrial fibrillation: A systematic review of age/gender differences and cardiovascular outcomes. International Journal of Cardiology. 2015;**191**:172-177. DOI: 10.1016/j.ijcard.2015.05.011

[49] Go A, Hylek E, Philips K, Chang Y, Henault L, Selby J, et al. Prevalence of diagnosed atrial fibrillation in adults: National implications for rhythm management and stroke prevention: The Anticoagulation and Risk Factors in Atrial Fibrillation (ATRIA) Study. Journal of the American Medical Association. 2001;**285**(18):2370-2375

[50] Wagstaff A, Overvad T, Lip G, Lane D. Is female sex a risk factor for stroke and thromboembolism in patients with atrial fibrillation? A systematic review and meta-analysis. QJM. 2014;**107**(12):955-967

[51] Defaye P, Dournaux F, Mouton E. Prevalence of supraventricular arrhythmias from the automated analysis of data stored in the DDD pacemakers of 617 patients: The AIDA study. The AIDA Multicenter Study Group. Automatic interpretation for

diagnosis assistance. Pacing and Clinical Electrophysiology. 1998;**21**(1 Pt 2): 250-255

[52] Garrigue S, Cazeau S, Ritter P, Lazarus A, Gras D, Mugica J. Incidence of atrial arrhythmia in patients with long term dual-chamber pacemakers. Contribution of the Holter function of pacemakers. Archives des Maladies du Coeur et des Vaisseaux. 1996;**89**(7):873-881

[53] Savelieva I, Camm AJ. Clinical relevance of silent atrial fibrillation: Prevalence, prognosis, quality of life, and management. Journal of Interventional Cardiac Electrophysiology. 2000;**4**(2):369-382

[54] Chugh SS, Havmoeller R, Narayanan K, Singh D, Rienstra M, Benjamin EJ, et al. Worldwide epidemiology of atrial fibrillation: A global burden of disease 2010 study. Circulation. 2014;**129**(8):837-847. DOI: 10.1161/CIRCULATIONAHA.113.005119

[55] Thrall G, Lane D, Carroll D, Lip GY. Quality of life in patients with atrial fibrillation: A systematic review. The American Journal of Medicine. 2006;**119**(5):448.e1-448.19

[56] McCabe PJ. Self-management of atrial fibrillation: A new frontier for nursing research. Progress in Cardiovascular Nursing. 2008;**23**(1):37-40

[57] McCabe PJ. What patients want and need to know about atrial fibrillation. Journal of Multidisciplinary Healthcare. 2011;**4**:413-419. DOI: 10.2147/JMDH.S19315

[58] Peterson ED, Ho PM, Barton M, Beam C, Burgess LH, Casey DE Jr, et al. ACC/AHA/AACVPR/AAFP/ANA concepts for clinician-patient shared accountability in performance measures: A report of the American College of Cardiology/American Heart Association task force on performance measures. Circulation. 2014;**130**(22):1984-1994. DOI: 10.1161/CIRC.0000000000000139

[59] Donal E, Colette E, Hubert A. Could transthoracic echocardiography results be convincing enough to impact the management of atrial fibrillation? Echocardiography. 2016;**33**(5):672-673. DOI: 10.1111/echo.13201

[60] Donal E, Lip GY, Galderisi M, Goette A, Shah D, Marwan M, et al. EACVI/EHRA Expert Consensus Document on the role of multi-modality imaging for the evaluation of patients with atrial fibrillation. European Heart Journal Cardiovascular Imaging. 2016;**17**(4):355-383. DOI: 10.1093/ehjci/jev354

[61] Fabritz L, Guasch E, Antoniades C, Bardinet I, Benninger G, Betts TR, et al. Expert consensus document: Defining the major health modifiers causing atrial fibrillation: A roadmap to underpin personalized prevention and treatment. Nature Reviews. Cardiology. 2016;**13**(4):230-237. DOI: 10.1038/nrcardio.2015

[62] Deneer VH, van Hemel NM. Is antiarrhythmic treatment in the elderly different? A review of the specific changes. Drugs & Aging. 2011;**28**(8):617-633. DOI: 10.2165/11591680-000000000-00000

[63] Fabritz L, Kirchhof P. Predictable and less predictable unwanted cardiac drugs effects: Individual pre-disposition and transient precipitating factors. Basic & Clinical Pharmacology & Toxicology. 2010;**106**(3):263-268. DOI: 10.1111/j.1742-7843.2010.00547.x

[64] Magnusson P, Kovi H, Mattsson G. A protocol for a prospective observational study using chest and

thumb ECG: Transient ECG assessment in stroke evaluation (TEASE) in Sweden. BMJ Open. 2018;**8**:019933

[65] Coala. The RedHeart Study: Coala. 2018. Available from: https://www.coalalife.com/english-news/2018/5/29/the-red-heart-study-z6x7e [Accessed: November 29, 2018]

[66] Bergman S Jr, Hoffler G, Johnson R. Evaluation of the electromechanical properties of the cardiovascular system. Houston, Texas: NASA. 1974. Available from: https://ntrs.nasa.gov/search.jsp?R=19750006321 [Accessed: November 29, 2018]

[67] Hassan S, Turner P. Systolic time intervals: A review of the method in the non-invasive investigation of cardiac function in health, disease and clinical pharmacology. Postgraduate Medical Journal. 1983;**59**(693):423-434